the breast cancer cookbook

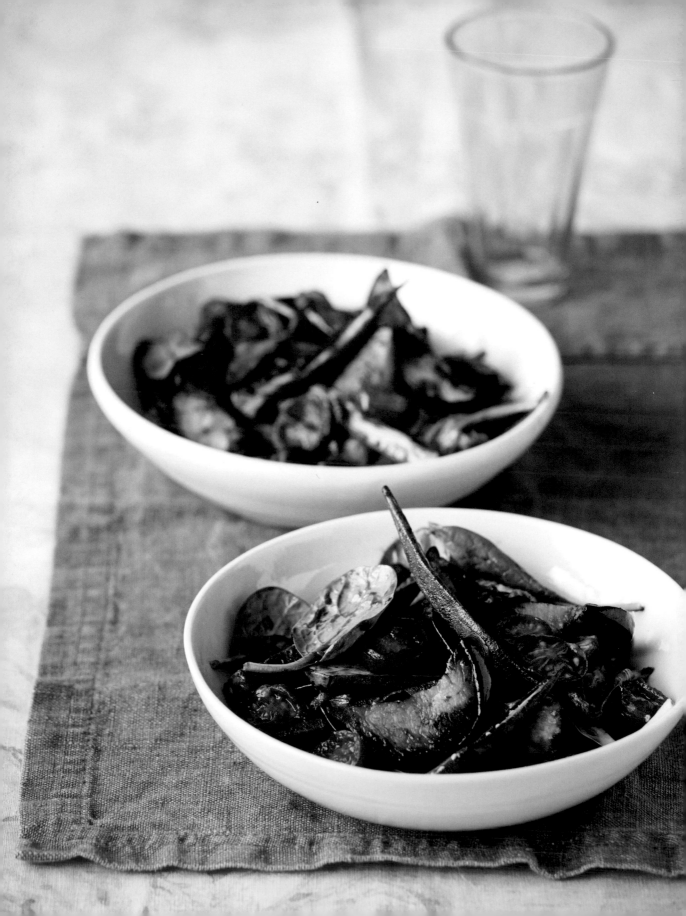

the breast cancer cookbook

*Over 100 easy recipes for cancer prevention
and to boost health during and after treatment*

Professor Mohammed Keshtgar

Consultant Breast Cancer Specialist, The Royal Free

with Dr Claire Robertson
and Dr Miriam Dwek

Recipes by Emily Jonzen
Photography by Jan Baldwin

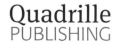
Quadrille
PUBLISHING

Recipe notes

All recipes have been analysed for their calorie, total fat, saturated fat, sugar and salt contents per 100g and per portion to ensure they are appropriate for inclusion in a healthy balanced diet.

All spoon measures are level unless otherwise stated:
1 tsp = 5ml spoon;
1 tbsp = 15ml spoon.

Please use fresh herbs and freshly ground pepper unless otherwise suggested.

Use medium eggs unless otherwise suggested. Anyone who is pregnant or in a vulnerable health group should avoid recipes that use raw egg whites or lightly cooked eggs.

If using the zest of citrus fruit, buy unwaxed fruit.

Timings are guidelines for fan-assisted ovens. If you are using a conventional oven, set your oven temperature approximately 15°C (1 Gas mark) higher. Use an oven thermometer to check the temperature.

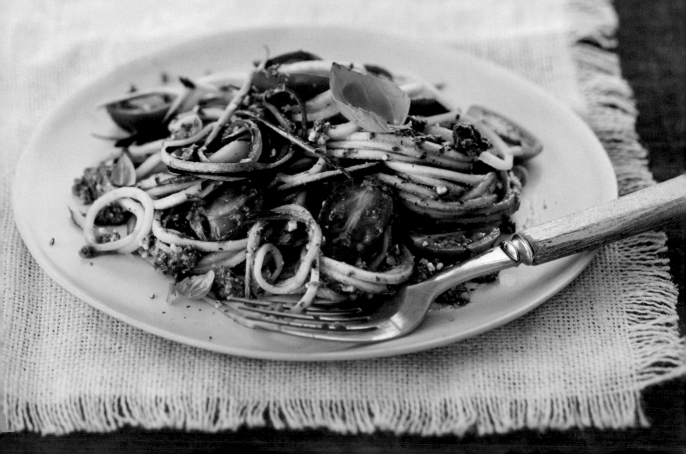

Contents

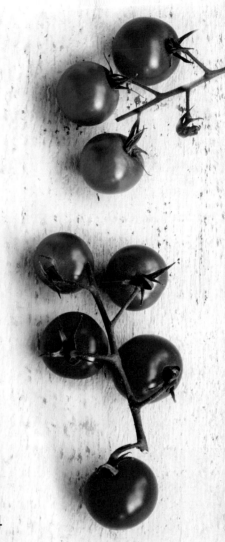

Introduction

You may be reading this book because you have been diagnosed with breast cancer, either recently or a while ago, or you may feel that you have a higher risk of developing it, perhaps because you have one or more relatives with breast cancer. Or you may be fit and well and simply are concerned about your health in some way. I was motivated to write this book in collaboration with my colleagues as I have become increasingly convinced that diet and lifestyle are contributing factors to the development of cancer.

Over the years, I have met and treated countless women, and some men, with breast cancer. In my experience, when a patient is informed of their breast cancer diagnosis, after a short period of getting over the shock of the news, the majority would like to take an active role in their treatment. They find loss of control difficult to bear and they would like to regain that control. I am asked to advise them on what they can do to help them fight the disease. Diet and lifestyle are two aspects that they can modify immediately, and with relative ease.

Many feel empowered to take responsibility for themselves. This also helps them to go into fight mode and psychologically feel better about themselves and their treatment. This experience is coupled with the fact that there have been major advances in the effective treatment of breast cancer. Being diagnosed with the disease is not all doom and gloom and the majority of our patients make a full recovery after treatment.

Approximately 30% of cancers and their sequelae are influenced by five behavioural risk factors: dietary intake, high body mass index, low fruit and vegetable intake, lack of physical activity, tobacco and alcohol use. No single factor is causal or protective, and many factors interplay in some way.

Eating and drinking are an integral part of our lives. We are what we eat and our lifestyle can contribute to our general well-being and also to the development of cancer. We are also able to modify our diet and therefore alter the risk of developing cancer, including breast cancer. Changes in dietary patterns are not only related to a reduction in the risk of developing breast cancer, there is also evidence that breast cancer recurrence rates are reduced and survival is improved when patients diagnosed and treated for breast cancer adopt a healthy lifestyle.

It is estimated that as many as 9% of cancer cases may be prevented by individuals changing their diet. Research also suggests that about 5% could be avoided by maintaining a healthy body weight. Of course, it takes time to change your diet, certainly for you to be content with that change, and for it to become lasting. If, for example, your diet has been low in fruit and vegetables, yet high in sugary foods such as cakes and biscuits, and you are looking to reverse that balance, it will take time for your appetite to adapt… but adapt it will, if you are motivated and persistent. It follows that the consequent improvement to your health and well-being will also take time.

'Approximately 30% of cancers are influenced by behavioural risk factors, including dietary intake, being overweight, low fruit and vegetable intake, lack of physical activity, tobacco and alcohol use.'

What is breast cancer?

Normal tissues are made up of cells of different types that are arranged to form an organ, such as a breast. It is the DNA that controls what happens in the cell. When the DNA changes (a process called mutation), it leads to cells starting to grow out of control and ultimately results in cancer.

Breast cancer is by far the commonest cancer in women. Worldwide, more than 1.5 million women are diagnosed with breast cancer every year. The majority of women develop breast cancer after their menopause, but about two out of every ten patients are under 50 years of age. The risk of developing breast cancer for a woman who lives to 85 years of age in the UK is currently 1 in 8. Thanks to significant developments in medicine and the biomedical sciences, more than 85% of the women diagnosed with breast cancer remain alive and well 5 years after their diagnosis.

Breast cancer risk factors

Breast cancer is a multi-factorial disease and although its causes and natural history remain unclear, epidemiological research indicates that genetic, biological, environmental, dietary and lifestyle aspects are amongst the risk factors for the disease.

Key risk factors include the individual's reproductive history. For example, exposure to a greater number of menstrual cycles, that is to say early-age onset of menstruation and late-age onset of menopause, as well as having fewer children, are risk factors. Being overweight and consumption of alcohol are also amongst the risk factors. The underlying reason for this increased risk is the exposure to the female sex hormone oestrogen; this hormone is known to bind to a receptor molecule in breast cells and drive cell division. Increased cell division increases the chance of an individual developing breast cancer. Preventing long-term exposure to oestrogen reduces the risk of breast cancer.

HRT (hormone replacement therapy) involves taking female sex hormones to replace hormones that your ovaries no longer produce after menopause. It is mainly taken in order to reduce the symptoms of menopause like hot flushes and lack of energy. Taking HRT increases the risk of developing breast and ovarian cancer. The longer you take HRT, the more your breast cancer risk increases. The good news is that if you are already taking HRT and have decided to stop, your risk of cancer development will revert back to normal within 5 years of stopping it.

Aside from reproductive history, inheriting a faulty (mutated) gene is responsible for approximately 5–10% of all breast cancers. The most common of these are the BRCA1 and BRCA2 genes. If you have a faulty gene, it doesn't mean you'll definitely develop breast cancer, but you are at a higher risk. Out of every 100 women with a faulty gene, between 50 and 85 of them will develop breast cancer in their lifetime.

Gene testing, which is done by a blood test, can be offered to you, if you have a high-risk family history of breast or ovarian cancer. This can include close relatives of women with a faulty gene, and women with a strong family history of breast cancer. It is preferable that a living family member with breast or ovarian cancer is available for gene testing, however it is possible to do the test if this is not the case.

'Breast cancer risk factors include exposure to a greater number of menstrual cycles, taking HRT, having fewer children, lack of breast feeding, being overweight, consumption of alcohol and inheriting a faulty gene.'

If you are found to have a faulty gene, the options include undergoing preventative mastectomy, as was the case with Angelina Jolie, which significantly raised the public awareness about gene testing. The other options include prevention by the use of anti-hormone drugs such as Tamoxifen. Alternatively, you may choose to opt for regular yearly check ups and undergo active surveillance.

Treatment for breast cancer

If you have been diagnosed with breast cancer, various treatments may be offered to you, depending on the features related to you and your cancer. These treatment options include surgery, which may involve removing the lump (lumpectomy) or the whole breast (mastectomy).

Radiotherapy involves using high energy x-rays to kill cancer cells, and some patients may receive this treatment after breast surgery. It involves coming to hospital on a daily basis for up to 4–5 weeks and receiving the treatment by lying under the x-ray delivery machine for a few minutes per treatment.

Hormonal treatment works by giving a drug that prevents the female sex hormone oestrogen from stimulating cancer cells. This treatment is recommended if the cancer is hormone responsive, which can be checked under the microscope after surgery.

'Over the years, there have been significant advances in the diagnosis and treatment of breast cancer. These include advances in surgery, radiotherapy, anti-hormone medications and chemotherapy.'

Chemotherapy is the use of drugs to kill cancer cells and there are a number of chemotherapy drugs that can be used alone or in combination for the treatment of breast cancer.

This treatment is usually delivered intravenously at three-weekly intervals (cycles) and is extremely effective. Many individuals tolerate the treatment well and are able to eat normally during chemotherapy, however a small minority may suffer one or more side effects that can impact on their eating. So let's explore this in more detail.

Chemotherapy can affect the appetite. This may happen soon after the delivery of the drugs and may be associated with feeling sick (nausea) and vomiting, which can be controlled by anti-sickness medication. These symptoms usually improve within a few days of each treatment. It is important to eat regularly (albeit small portions) and keep well hydrated by drinking plenty of water.

The other possible side effect of chemotherapy is soreness of the mouth, which can lead to discomfort during eating. It may be helpful to avoid consuming spicy, acidic and very hot foods until the underlying problem is settled. Some patients have reported discomfort whilst swallowing owing to this problem and the use of soups and semi-solid foods would be helpful in this situation.

Some patients who receive chemotherapy may experience a change in their taste sensation, finding that most of their usual foods taste somewhat bland. This is due to the effect of chemotherapy on tastebuds. The inclusion of strongly flavoured foods during this period may help to overcome the problem.

Chemotherapy can also affect bowel habits, resulting in either diarrhoea or constipation. Loose motions may occur due to the effect of the chemotherapy drugs on the lining of the gut, and it is imperative that you drink plenty of fluid to avoid dehydration during this period.

On the other hand, constipation can happen due to the lack of physical activity and also as a side effect of some of the supportive drugs, like painkillers and anti-sickness medication. Drinking plenty of fluid and eating high-fibre foods such as fruit and vegetables should help to alleviate this problem.

Finally, you may be surprised to know that most patients are inclined to put on, rather than lose, a bit of weight during chemotherapy. This is due to a combination of factors, including reduced mobility and exercise, comfort eating and as a side effect to the family of drugs called steroids, which lead to fluid retention in the body and increase the appetite. It is important to stick to a well-balanced diet, as described in this book, during this period. Most patients are able to shed the excess weight easily after completion of their chemotherapy, by increasing their daily physical activity and continuing to eat a healthy diet.

Diet and lifestyle influences

Global studies exploring geographical differences in breast cancer incidence have taught us a lot about diet and lifestyle influences. For example, in Northern Europe the percentage of breast cancer cases is about three times higher than in Eastern Asia. Studies of populations that migrate from areas with

'Chemotherapy is the use of drugs to kill cancer cells. Many individuals tolerate the treatment well and are able to eat normally, however a minority suffer a few side effects that can impact on their eating. There are effective ways to overcome these side effects.'

'Global studies exploring geographical differences in the incidence of breast cancer clearly suggest that dietary, lifestyle and environmental factors contribute to the risk of developing the disease.'

low breast cancer risk (such as Japan) to areas of high breast cancer risk (the US, for instance) have shown that the risk of developing the disease increases to approximately that of the host nation within a few generations. Clearly, this suggests that dietary, lifestyle and environmental factors are contributing factors to the risk of developing breast cancer.

Moreover, epidemiological evidence suggests that the Mediterranean diet could reduce the risk of breast cancer. A comprehensive study of approximately 330,000 women in 10 European countries over an 11-year period ending in the year 2000 showed that adherence to a Mediterranean diet excluding alcohol was related to a modest risk reduction of breast cancer in post-menopausal women.

Our own research is focusing on the effects of diet and lifestyle on the recurrence of breast cancer. We are coordinating the largest dietary study to date of breast cancer patients within the UK. The study is called DietCompLyf and includes over 3,000 patients from 56 NHS hospitals. We expect that the study will start to yield results in the very near future.

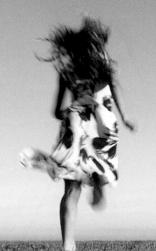
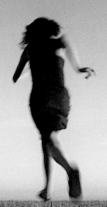

Body weight There is a definite link between body mass index (BMI) and breast cancer. Being overweight and having excess weight around the stomach (central adiposity) is linked to the incidence of post-menopausal breast cancer. Weight gain after the age of 20 and high weight gain during mid adulthood also increase the risk of breast cancer. The association seems to be more pronounced for breast cancer diagnosed before or at the age of 50, so it is important to keep fit and avoid weight gain during this period.

Without doubt, eating a balanced diet and keeping active will help to maintain a healthy weight and reduce the risk of breast cancer.

Physical activity Regular physical activity can improve health by helping to control weight, reducing the risk of heart disease and keeping the blood pressure steady. It also promotes psychological well-being by increasing the levels of endorphins (the 'happy hormones') in the body.

Physical activity also helps to keep bones strong and healthy. This holds true particularly with weight-bearing exercises like walking and light jogging. This type of activity is particularly useful for breast cancer patients who are on the specialised anti-hormone medications known as aromatase inhibitors, the long-term use of which can predispose to osteoporosis.

Although this is a difficult area to investigate, several studies have confirmed the link between physical activity and reduced risk of cancer, in particular breast and bowel cancer. The indication that a high level of physical activity reduces the risk of post-menopausal breast cancer is particularly notable.

The Department of Health recommends moderate-intensity physical activity for at least 30 minutes, five or more days a week, or at least 20 minutes of high-intensity exercise for three or more days a week.

Alcohol consumption Alcohol consumption has been linked to an increase in both the risk of developing breast cancer and the likelihood of breast cancer recurrence. This is independent of the type of alcoholic drink consumed and menopausal status. Since the early 1980s, numerous studies have examined this link.

'Eating a balanced diet and doing regular physical activity not only reduces the risk of developing breast cancer, but also lessens the risk of bowel cancer and heart disease, and improves your bone health.'

Even for light drinkers, there appears to be a moderate increased risk. That risk increases with the volume of alcohol consumed. For women who have three or more alcoholic drinks per day there is a 40–50% elevated risk of breast cancer.

The exact mechanism by which alcohol raises breast cancer risk is not clear. Alcohol probably functions by a 'secondary effect', i.e. it adversely affects the ability of the liver to remove oestrogen from the blood system, which leads to a rise in blood oestrogen levels. As oestrogen can stimulate the growth of breast cells, this may raise the risk of breast cancer. Also, breakdown products of alcohol may lead to mutations in cells by affecting proteins that usually protect and repair cellular DNA.

Moderate alcohol intake may protect against cardiovascular disease and it is pertinent to remember that cardiovascular disease is a considerably greater risk to women than breast cancer. Once a patient has developed breast cancer, however, there is evidence that alcohol consumption may not be advisable.

'Alcohol consumption has been linked to an increase in both the risk of developing breast cancer and the likelihood of breast cancer recurrence. Once a patient has developed breast cancer, there is evidence to indicate that alcohol consumption is not advisable.'

Specific dietary associations with breast cancer

We know that dietary and lifestyle choices may help to prevent breast cancer and its recurrence, and may also prevent the development of other diseases. In recent years, there have been many reports in the press about the role certain foods play in both the development of cancer and protection from it, not all of them substantiated by plausible research studies, so let's explore these in more detail.

Dietary fats There is some evidence that both the total amount of fat and the amount of saturated fat consumed in the diet are associated with both the risk of developing post-menopausal breast cancer and poorer survival after a breast cancer diagnosis. The sources of such fat are butter, margarine and cooking oil, as well as the fats from meats of various sources and 'hidden fats' in cakes, biscuits and snack foods.

Sugars and carbs In recent years, some studies have suggested that the consumption of carbohydrates has been related to breast cancer risk, however the analysis of all studies performed in this field does not support this and, overall, the conclusion is that there is no association between carbohydrate intake and breast cancer risk.

Dairy products

Despite many misleading media reports, there is no scientific evidence to support the idea that milk or dairy products increase breast cancer risk, or affect prognosis after a breast cancer diagnosis. This misconception stems from the observation that the incidence of breast cancer is low in countries like China where the consumption of dairy foods is low. However, researchers believe that the low incidence is mainly due to other lifestyle differences.

As milk is a complex food that includes vitamins, minerals, carbohydrates, fats and proteins, dairy-based foods are very difficult to study either in the laboratory or in population studies. Some laboratory studies have suggested that certain proteins in the milk can stimulate cell growth but these results have not been replicated in humans. In contrast, high levels of intake of dairy products have been shown to be associated with a reduced risk of pre-menopausal breast cancer. As dairy products are an important source of calcium, which is essential for bone health, moderate consumption of low-fat dairy produce is advised.

Meat intake

The results of scientific studies concerning the consumption of meat products and poultry are inconsistent and further research is required. Current evidence suggests that the consumption of non-processed meat in moderation as a part of a balanced diet is quite safe (see page 18).

Fruit, vegetables and dietary fibre

Vegetables and fruit may well have a preventative effect against cancer, as they are rich in antioxidants and vitamins, including vitamins C, E and folate; they are also an important source of dietary fibre. An antioxidant prevents a chemical process called oxidation in which oxygen molecules are joined with other chemicals to create reactive products. These reactive products have been shown to cause gene damage in cells and such damage may ultimately lead to cancer development.

Despite this clear evidence of protective effects, the evidence for decreased breast cancer risk based on the consumption of

'There is no evidence to suggest that the consumption of milk or dairy products increases breast cancer risk; the same holds true for meat products. Consuming lean meat in moderation as part of a balanced diet is deemed perfectly safe.'

fruit and vegetables is limited and further studies are needed. With regard to fibre, studies suggest that a diet rich in dietary fibre is likely to reduce the risk of developing breast cancer.

Phytoestrogens

One of the main foodstuffs consumed in high quantities in Eastern diets is soy. Examples of soy food include pulses and cereals, tofu, green vegetables and soya milk. These foods are enriched in plant chemicals, which have molecules similar to the female sex hormone oestrogen and are known as phytoestrogens. They can behave like human oestrogen and bind to receptors in cells, preventing naturally occurring oestrogen from binding. Because of this property, phytoestrogens are thought to have a protective role against breast cancer by preventing cancer cell growth.

Researchers have tried to establish if consumption of soy and fermented soy (e.g. tofu) is linked to a decreased risk of developing breast cancer, and whether this also relates to reduced breast cancer recurrence rates. There is some evidence to suggest that this is the case, in both Western and Eastern populations.

The picture is somewhat more complicated when a patient has already been diagnosed with breast cancer, as phytoestrogens have the potential to interfere with hormonal treatments which function by binding to the oestrogen receptor. There may still be a link between better survival after breast cancer and the consumption of foods containing soy, but further research is needed into this topic.

'Soy-rich foods including edamame beans, dried soya beans, tofu, miso and soya milk contain phytoestrogens, which have properties similar to the female sex hormone oestrogen. These are thought to have a protective effect against breast cancer by preventing cancer cell growth.'

Tea and coffee

Green tea, black tea and coffee are difficult to study as they contain varied ingredients and show batch-to-batch and geographical differences. There have been some animal studies which suggest that green tea extracts may combine with the breast cancer drug Tamoxifen and reduce side effects. Further research is required to confirm these results in humans and also to establish the effects of black tea and coffee in this regard.

Taking the above into consideration, we have prepared a guide to foods to eat more of, foods to eat in moderation and foods you should be cautious of. This is followed by a collection of recipes, which have been carefully devised, incorporating the current evidence to help you towards a healthy, well-balanced diet.

Moving towards a healthier diet and lifestyle

Diet and its effect on health is a complex subject. However limited an individual's diet may be, it will still involve a range of foods, which means a diverse intake of ingredients and nutrients at almost every single meal. From time to time, research studies may identify a potentially protective or causal relationship between a food or nutrient and a breast cancer outcome. There are often reports in the press suggesting that a specific food, food group or nutrient may increase or reduce your risk of cancer, but it is never that straightforward. It is more often the complex combination of several causal or protective factors that explains the outcome.

Understandably, anyone diagnosed with breast cancer is likely to react to media reports linking breast cancer to the intake of specific foods, but we need to be cautious about interpreting these reports and implementing dietary changes. In particular, cutting out specific foods can be detrimental if it leads to a deficiency of important nutrients. All too often we come across contradictory media reports presenting conflicting advice, just a few months apart.

We know that breast cancer and many other chronic diseases can be slowed and/or prevented by dietary and lifestyle modifications, but it is all about adopting and maintaining a healthy, balanced approach. The following advice is based on this premise:

Balance your diet Nutrition is vital for every cellular process in our bodies. Aim to eat a wide variety of food to ensure you are getting all the nutrients you need. Think about the ingredients you are choosing, and how they will influence your mood and health.

Stay in shape Reaching and maintaining a healthy weight is one of the most important goals for all. Evidence clearly highlights its importance as a means of preventing cancer and the progression of the disease.

Move more Exercise not only mitigates cancer risk through weight reduction, it can also lower levels of oestrogen in our bodies and modify the ways in which we physically store and process the foods we eat.

Enjoy your food Think about what you are going to eat, shop wisely (especially for fresh items), take the time to prepare your meals and, above all, enjoy what you eat.

Foods to eat more of...

These are foods that can offer significant health benefits, so it is worth looking to ensure you include them in your diet on a regular and, in most cases, frequent basis.

Fruit and veg Aim to include at least 5 portions (400g) from as diverse a range of produce as possible. Particularly good choices include the following:

· **Tomatoes** A powerful source of the antioxidant lycopene (particularly following cooking/processing), which gives tomatoes their redness and has the potential to inhibit breast cancer by stopping cancer cell growth.

· **Cruciferous veg** This food group, which includes broccoli, Brussels sprouts, cauliflower, kale and cabbage, is an excellent source of phytonutrients, which can help to prevent the formation of cancer cells and stop the spread of cancer.

· **Dark green leafy veg** Vibrant vegetables such as spinach, kale and beetroot leaves are loaded with folate, a B vitamin that strengthens your DNA and which can reduce cancer risk.

Wholegrain starchy staples Choose nutrient-rich quinoa, bulgar, spelt, brown rice, potatoes and wholegrain breads over their refined equivalents.

Beans and pulses These are an excellent source of vegetable protein. Vital for growth and development, protein is necessary to enable your body to repair any damage imposed by cancer treatments. In addition to protein, beans and pulses provide a range of other valuable nutrients, including calcium, iron and B vitamins.

Omega-3 rich oily fish Include fish such as salmon, sardines and mackerel in your diet once or twice each week to ensure you are getting omega-3 fatty acids. Apart from helping to decrease inflammation in the body, these foods can also provide a dietary source of vitamin D to promote calcium uptake by the bones.

Olive oil Make this your first choice for cooking and salad dressings. It is loaded with risk-reducing antioxidants and phytonutrients, and has a higher than typical monounsaturated fat content, which can prevent oxidation, the process which produces free radicals known to increase cancer risk.

Foods to eat in moderation…

Labelling any individual food as 'bad for you' or 'to be avoided' is misleading. The following foods have received a bad press from time to time but they are important sources of vital nutrients and merit inclusion in a balanced diet.

Red meat There have been many conflicting reports about the positive and negative effects of consuming red meat. A high-quality protein food, meat is also a great source of other valuable nutrients, especially B vitamins and minerals – notably zinc, iron and selenium. The haem-iron red meat provides is especially beneficial, as it is more easily absorbed than iron from plant sources, and can have a positive impact on energy levels.

On the downside, red meat (fattier cuts, in particular) tends to be high in saturated fats. Eaten in moderation, red meat can play an important role in a healthy diet. Our advice would be to choose leaner cuts, trim off excess fat and aim to keep your intake to an average maximum of 70–90g per day. You can easily achieve this by having some meat-free days during the week.

Always avoid over-cooking meat using a grill or barbecue, as this can produce heterocyclic amines (HCA) and polycyclic aromatic hydrocarbons (PAH), which may be carcinogenic.

Dairy foods These are great sources of protein and calcium, the mineral that is so vital for bone health. The calcium in dairy foods is more readily absorbed than it is from plant sources, and when consumed in high levels, is associated with greater excretion of dietary fat. Although dairy foods have relatively high levels of saturated fat, nutritional concerns are linked only to situations where their intake contributes to calorie excess (and therefore weight gain). Given that they are such important sources of micro-nutrients, we would recommend that dairy foods are consumed on a daily basis (unless, of course, you have a lactose intolerance). Look to gain the benefits from semi-skimmed milk, natural yogurt and fromage frais and limit your intake of high-fat cheeses, butter and cream.

Foods to be cautious of…

No single food is known to cause cancer to develop or to recur. Evidence, however, has identified some foods (and nutrients), which should be eaten in small proportions, or completely avoided, to minimise your risk. These include:

Alcohol As explained on pages 12–13, there is a link between alcohol intake and breast cancer. If you have been diagnosed with breast cancer, it is advisable to avoid (or minimise) alcohol.

Trans fatty acids The use of artificial sources of trans fatty acids increases total cholesterol and lowers the 'good' (HDL) cholesterol in the body, so they should therefore be avoided. Watch out for sources in:
- **ready-made biscuits, cakes and pastries** made with partially hydrogenated fats and oils
- **hard margarines**
- **meat products** such as burgers, kebabs, pies and pastries
- **fat spreads** made using partially hydrogenated oils
- **savoury snacks** such as potato crisps.

Sweets It is advisable to limit or avoid sources of refined sugar, particularly those that do not offer other useful nutrients, as their intake can be associated with high blood glucose levels and consequently elevated insulin concentrations, a known risk factor for breast cancer development.

Processed meats Some preservatives used in the production of processed meats, including bacon, ham and hot dogs, are thought (but not proven) to be carcinogenic. Aside from potential carcinogens, these products are generally high in saturated fat and salt, so it makes sense to limit their intake.

Breakfast

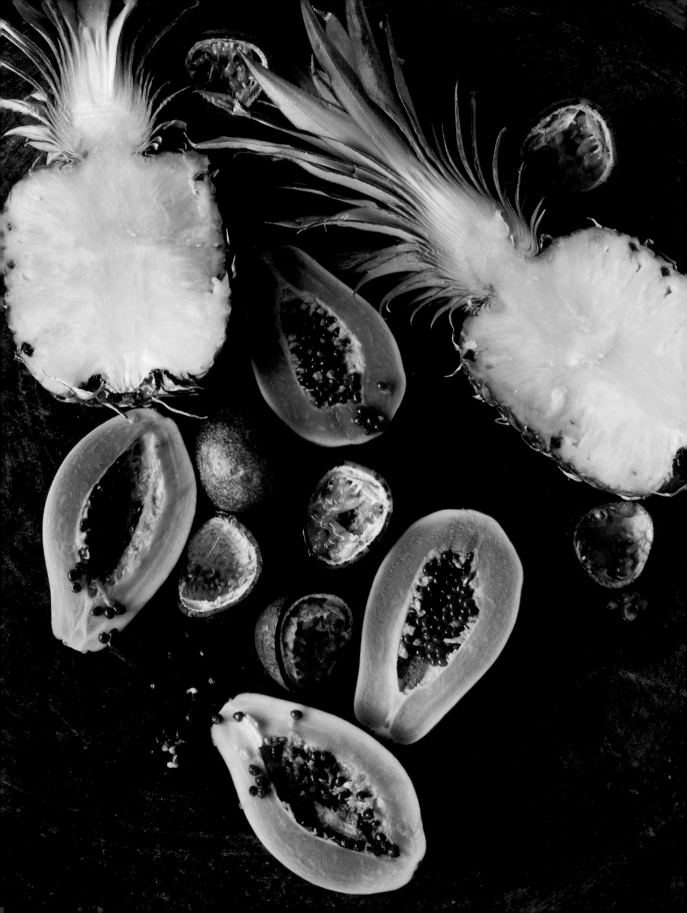

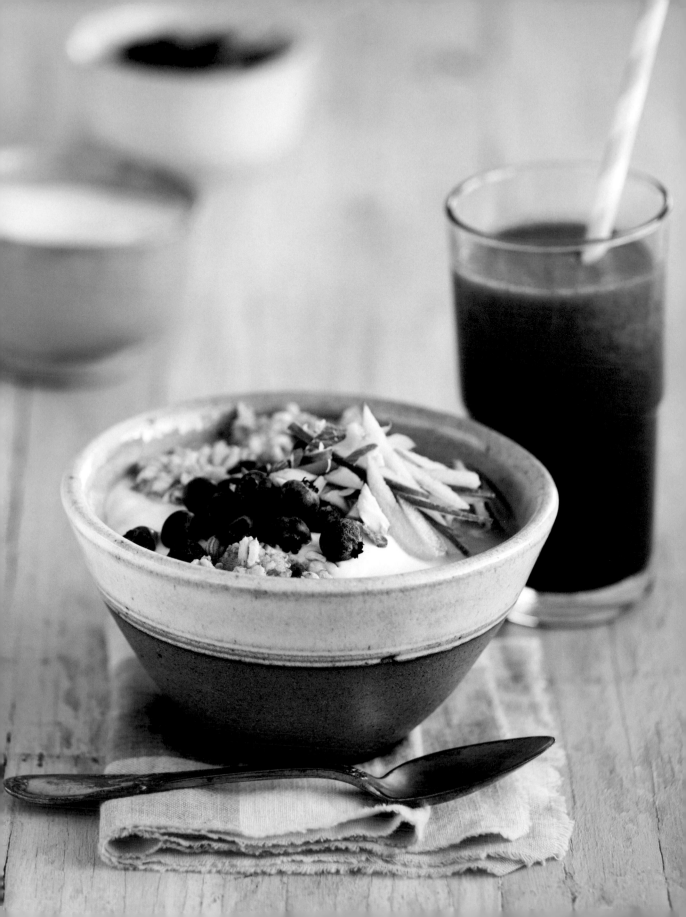

Bircher muesli
with apples and blueberries

Serves 4

120g jumbo oats

40g spelt flakes

200ml sugar-free cloudy
apple juice

350ml water

100g natural yogurt

2 sharp dessert apples,
such as Cox or Braeburn,
finely sliced or coarsely grated

100g blueberries

A pinch of ground cinnamon

2 tbsp raw almonds, roughly
chopped

This traditional Swiss muesli is more like a summer porridge than the muesli we are more familiar with. The grains are soaked to release the creaminess of the oats and served with natural yogurt and fresh fruit for a light breakfast.

Tip the oats and spelt flakes into a mixing bowl and pour on the apple juice and water. Cover and leave to soak in the fridge for 2 hours or overnight.

Spoon the soaked oats and spelt into serving bowls and top with the yogurt, apple, blueberries, cinnamon and chopped almonds.

Muesli with dried fruit, almonds and sunflower seeds

10–12 servings

400g jumbo oats

100g spelt flakes

75g raw almonds, roughly chopped

50g sunflower seeds

100g dried figs, finely chopped

100g dates, pitted and finely chopped

Making your own, delicious muesli couldn't be simpler. Once you try it you will wonder why you ever bought packets from the supermarket.

Preheat the oven to 160°C/Gas 3. Line 2 medium baking sheets with baking parchment and set aside.

Stir the oats, spelt flakes, almonds and sunflower seeds together and divide this mixture between the 2 trays, spreading it evenly. Bake for 12 minutes, or until the almonds are very lightly toasted, stirring once halfway through cooking. Remove from the oven and transfer to a big mixing bowl.

Stir through the dried figs, breaking up any large clumps of fruit as you go, and set aside to cool completely before storing in a large jar or plastic container. Enjoy with milk or yogurt for breakfast.

Apple and cinnamon porridge

Serves 4

200g jumbo oats

2 sharp dessert apples, such as Cox or Braeburn, peeled and coarsely grated

600ml semi-skimmed cow's milk or almond milk

400ml water

½ tsp ground cinnamon

With its enticing apple and warming spice flavours, this porridge will feel like a real treat on an icy morning.

Put all of the ingredients into a saucepan and place over a medium heat. Cook the porridge, stirring regularly, for about 6–8 minutes, until the oats are soft and the apple has broken down slightly.

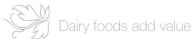 Dairy foods add value

After treatment for breast cancer, the risk of osteoporosis is increased. Although the hormone oestrogen is typically maligned because of its causal role in breast cancer, it also acts to strengthen bone by facilitating the uptake of calcium. As certain cancer treatments lead to a reduction of oestrogen levels and/or earlier initiation of menopause, the inclusion of dairy products within our diets has increasing importance. This warming porridge offers a sustaining breakfast that's packed with calcium. It also has the added nutritional benefits of fruit and a good proportion of soluble fibre to sustain hunger levels through the morning.

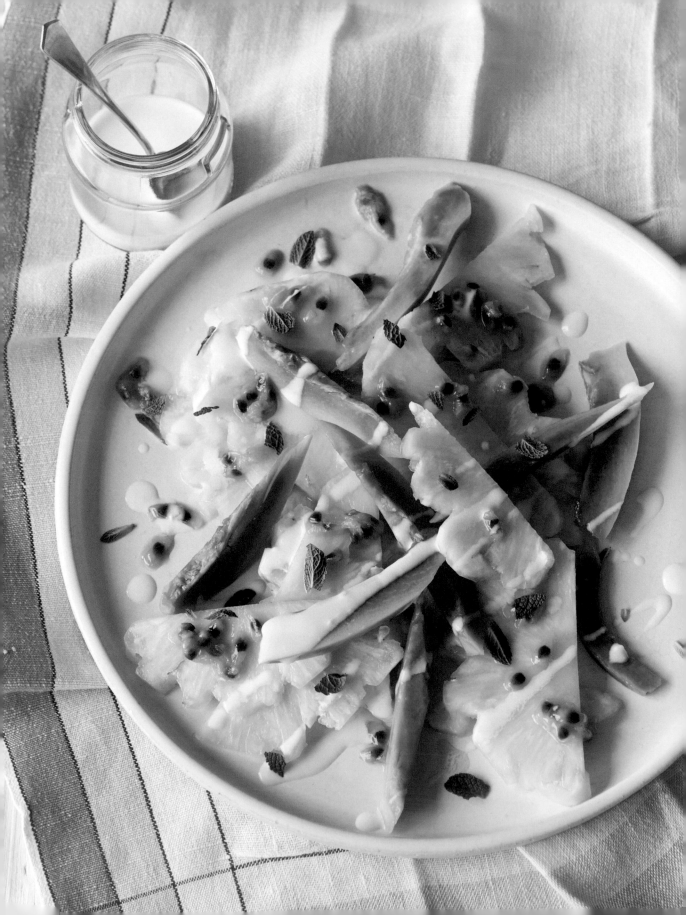

Tropical breakfast salad

Serves 4

2 small, ripe papayas, peeled, deseeded and sliced

1 small pineapple, peeled and sliced

2 passion fruit, halved

4 tbsp coconut cream

2 tbsp mint leaves, roughly chopped if large

For a super speedy and light breakfast, try this lively and indulgent combination. On a particularly hot day, this salad is wonderful served over crushed ice.

Lay the slices of papaya and pineapple out on a serving platter or individual plates and spoon over the passion fruit pulp. Drizzle with the coconut cream, scatter over the chopped mint and serve.

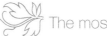 The most important meal of the day

Ideally, breakfast should provide 20–25% of both our recommended fruit and veg intake and our daily requirements for nutrients. Those of us who eat breakfast typically have a more nutritious, balanced diet overall compared to those who skip it. Without it, we can struggle to meet our daily micro-nutrient requirements and are more likely to resort to unhealthy snacks through the day to compensate. This can have an adverse impact on weight gain – a risk factor for the recurrence of breast cancer.

Boiled egg and nori asparagus soldiers

Serves 4

4 medium eggs, at room temperature

600g asparagus spears

1 tsp sunflower or rapeseed oil

2 tsp sesame seeds

2 tsp low-salt light soy sauce

1 nori sheet, crumbled into flakes

Spears of crunchy asparagus are the perfect healthy soldiers for dipping into a runny yolk. Teaming this combination with soy, sesame seeds and crushed nori makes it even more delicious.

Preheat the grill to high.

Bring a pan of water to the boil, then carefully lower the eggs into the water using a slotted spoon. Boil for 4 minutes for a runny yolk, 6 minutes for a semi-soft yolk and up to 9 minutes for a hard-boiled egg.

Meanwhile, snap off the woody ends of the asparagus and toss the spears in the oil, then lay them on a foil-lined baking sheet. Grill for 4 minutes, turning once.

Remove the baking sheet from the grill and sprinkle the sesame seeds and soy sauce over the asparagus. Grill for a further minute to toast the seeds; the asparagus should be burnished but tender with a little bite within.

Remove the eggs from the water with a slotted spoon and remove the tops of the shells with a knife. Place in egg cups. Sprinkle the asparagus soldiers with the nori flakes and dip away.

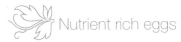 Nutrient rich eggs

Eggs are a good concentrated source of nutrients, providing all of the essential amino acids, all of the vitamins, except vitamin C, several important minerals and the powerful antioxidant selenium. In the past, negative press reports have linked eggs to high dietary cholesterol intake but it is now understood that the cholesterol we derive from consuming carbohydrate foods has more effect on our blood cholesterol level. Eggs are particularly valuable when your appetite is depleted. Served with asparagus dipping soldiers, they are the complete health-giving small meal to stimulate the appetite.

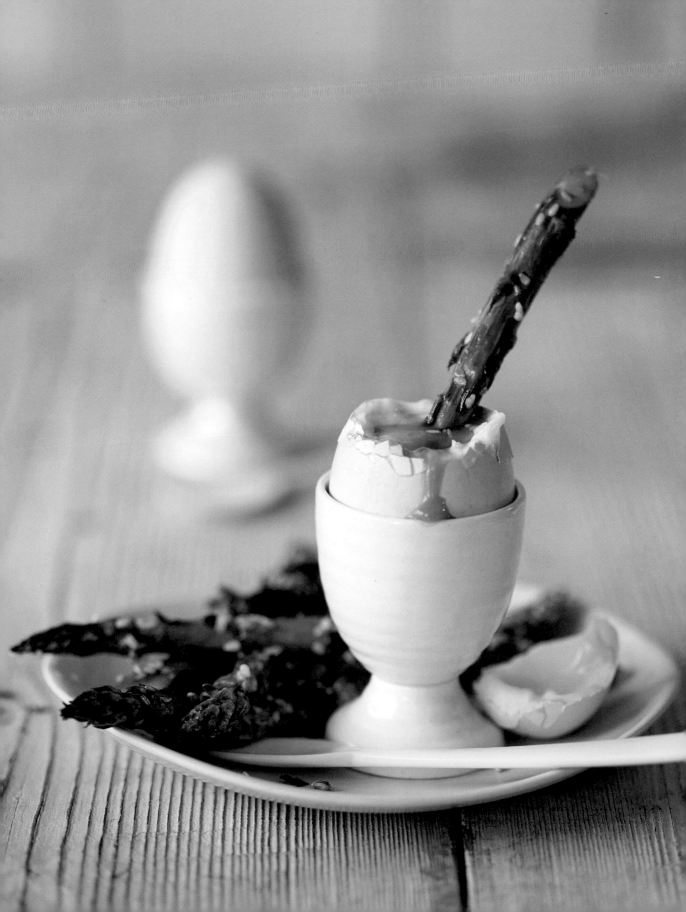

Home-baked beans on toast

Serves 4

2 tsp olive oil

1 onion, peeled and finely chopped

2 garlic cloves, peeled and crushed

2 tsp smoked paprika

1 tsp thyme leaves

2 tbsp tomato purée

400g can tomatoes

400g can cannellini beans or pinto beans, drained

1 tsp maple syrup

4 slices of bread

4 tbsp natural yogurt or low-fat crème fraîche

Homemade baked beans are infinitely tastier and more nutritious than their gloopy, sugar-saturated canned equivalent. These silky beans in a smoky tomato sauce are perfect for a hearty breakfast or brunch.

Heat the olive oil in a large saucepan over a medium-low heat. Add the onion and fry gently, stirring regularly, for 5 minutes until softened and golden, adding a little water if necessary. Stir in the garlic, smoked paprika, thyme and tomato purée and fry the mixture, stirring all the time, for a further 2 minutes until fragrant.

Meanwhile, blitz the tomatoes in a food processor until fine. Add to the saucepan and simmer for 10 minutes until slightly reduced.

Now add the beans and maple syrup and continue to simmer for 5 minutes. At this point, the sauce should be reduced and thick.

In the meantime, toast the slices of bread.

Serve the beans on the hot toast with a dollop of natural yogurt or crème fraîche.

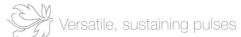 Versatile, sustaining pulses

Beans and other pulses are an economical and versatile food that offers a filling vegetarian alternative to meat. Canned pulses are a convenient fast food that can be added to soups and salads, blitzed to make dips or used to extend meat dishes. Relatively low in calories, yet satisfying, they are particularly useful if you have breast cancer as weight gain is a common consequence of treatment, and a key concern – due to its link with the risk of recurrence.

Baked feta eggs
with tomatoes, kale and dukkah

Serves 4

1 tsp olive oil

2 garlic cloves, peeled and crushed

4 spring onions, roughly sliced

100g kale, tough central stalk discarded, roughly chopped and rinsed

200g chopped tomatoes (fresh or canned)

4 medium eggs

60g light feta cheese

2 tsp dukkah (see right)

This easy-to-prepare, deeply savoury concoction makes for an unusual weekend brunch. Dukkah is a tasty Egyptian spiced nut and seed mix – try making your own (see below) and keeping it in a jar to sprinkle over salads and soups.

Preheat the oven to 180°C/Gas 4. Have a kettle filled with freshly boiled water and a roasting tin ready.

Heat the olive oil in a large frying pan over a medium heat. When it is hot, add the garlic and spring onions and fry for a couple of minutes, stirring frequently, until softened and golden. Add the kale and fry for a minute, until lightly wilted. Stir in the tomatoes and allow to bubble for a minute, then remove from the heat.

Spoon the kale mixture into 4 ramekins and make a dip in the centre of each. Crack an egg into each hollow, crumble over the feta and sprinkle with dukkah.

Stand the ramekins in the roasting tray and place in the oven. With the oven door ajar, carefully pour boiled water from the kettle into the roasting tin until it comes halfway up the sides of the ramekins. Close the oven door and bake for 12–15 minutes, until the egg whites are set but the yolks are still lovely and runny. Serve immediately.

Dukkah To make your own, lightly toast 50g almonds, 40g sesame seeds and 1 tbsp each coriander, cumin and sesame seeds in a heavy-based pan until fragrant, then grind to a coarse powder.

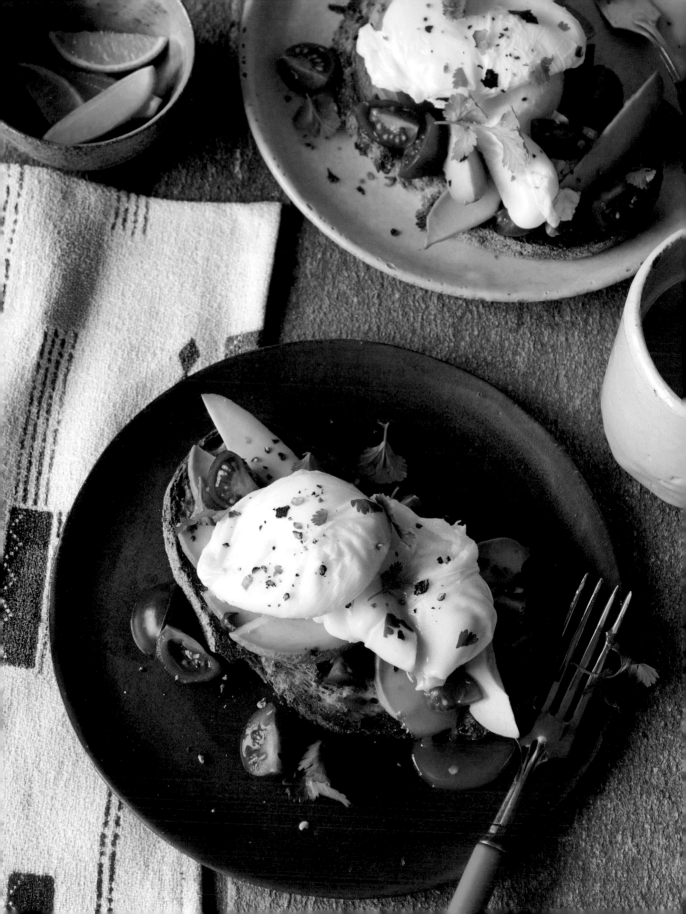

Mexican eggs

Serves 2

4 very fresh medium eggs, refrigerated

60g cherry tomatoes, quartered

1 avocado, halved, stoned, peeled and sliced

Juice of ½ lime

2 tbsp coriander leaves, roughly chopped

A pinch of dried chilli flakes (optional)

2 slices of sourdough or other rustic bread

Freshly ground black pepper

This bright and sunny breakfast sings with vibrant flavour. Be sure to seek out avocados at their peak of ripeness – to fully appreciate their creamy flavour.

For the poached eggs, fill a non-stick frying pan with a 4cm depth of water and bring to a simmer. Crack the eggs into a small bowl or ramekins and tip them, one at a time, into the water. Allow to simmer gently for 3 minutes, then carefully remove with a slotted spoon and drain on kitchen paper.

Meanwhile, in a bowl, toss together the cherry tomatoes, avocado, lime juice, most of the coriander and the chilli flakes, if using, and set aside.

Toast the bread and place a slice on each warmed plate. Spoon on the avocado mix, then top with the poached eggs, allowing two per person. Sprinkle with the remaining coriander, a little pepper and an extra touch of chilli, if required.

Quinoa, flax and chia seed bread

Makes 12–14 slices

150g wholemeal plain flour, plus extra to dust

150g quinoa flakes

2 tbsp milled flax seeds

2 tbsp chia seeds

2 tsp baking powder

A pinch of mineral salt

2 tbsp olive oil, plus a little extra to oil

1 medium egg, beaten

About 200ml tepid water

This fairly dense bread, with its slightly cracked crust, may not win any beauty prizes but it is brimming with flavour and nourishment. The slight nuttiness makes it a perfect breakfast loaf – enjoy with almond butter or a little honey.

Preheat the oven to 200°C/Gas 6. Lightly oil a 450g loaf tin and dust with a little flour.

Sift the wholemeal flour into a large mixing bowl and add any bran left in the sieve. Stir through the quinoa flakes, flax seeds, chia seeds, baking powder and salt and make a well in the centre.

Pour the olive oil, egg and 200ml water into the well and mix to form a fairly firm dough. If it looks a little dry, add another 1–2 tbsp water. Form a rough loaf shape and place in the prepared tin.

Bake for 40–45 minutes, until slightly risen and golden. To check that it is cooked, carefully remove the loaf from the tin and tap the underside. If it sounds hollow, it is cooked. Leave to cool slightly before slicing and serving.

Seeds: little nutrient powerhouses

Like nuts, seeds have numerous nutritional benefits. Although they have a high fat content, 75-80% of their fat is healthy unsaturated fats. An excellent source of omega-3s and omega-6s, they also provide soluble fibre, phytochemicals and plant sterols, which are deemed to protect against many non-communicable diseases, including cancer. Adding seeds to bread is a great way of improving the nutritional status of your loaf – as well as its texture.

Banana bread muffins

Makes 12

4 very ripe medium bananas

4 medium eggs, beaten

50g unsalted nut butter

4 tbsp vegetable oil

75g raisins

50g ground almonds

150g wholemeal flour

1 tsp baking powder

½ tsp ground cinnamon

These muffins are great to have as an instant standby nutritious breakfast. Ideal for freezing, simply defrost them and warm through briefly to return them to their just-baked glory.

Preheat the oven to 180°C/Gas 4 and line a 12-hole muffin tray with paper muffin cases.

Put the bananas, eggs, nut butter, oil and raisins into a food processor and blend for 2–3 minutes, until the bananas and raisins have broken down and the mixture is creamy and mousse-like.

Sift the remaining ingredients into a large mixing bowl, adding any bran and almonds left in the sieve, then fold in the wet ingredient mix until just combined.

Using an ice-cream scoop or tablespoon, divide the mixture between the muffin cases. Bake for 15 minutes, or until risen, golden, and a skewer inserted into the centre comes out clean. Allow to cool slightly and serve warm, or at room temperature.

The muffins will keep in an airtight container for up to 3 days.

Oat and spelt soda bread

Makes 16 slices

425g wholemeal spelt flour,
plus extra to dust

1 tsp bicarbonate of soda

A pinch of mineral salt

75g jumbo rolled oats

4 tbsp sunflower seeds

450g natural yogurt

1 tbsp clear honey

1 tbsp lemon juice

No kneading, rising or proving – soda bread has to be one of the simplest, and most delicious things to bake. Spelt flour lends a light nuttiness to this traditional Irish loaf.

Preheat the oven to 200°C/Gas 6 and dust a non-stick baking sheet with flour. Sift the flour, bicarbonate of soda and salt into a large mixing bowl and add any bran left in the sieve. Stir through the oats and sunflower seeds and make a well in the centre.

Mix the yogurt with the honey and lemon juice, pour into the centre of the well and quickly stir to form a sticky dough. Using lightly floured hands, carefully bring the dough together into a loose round and transfer to the prepared baking sheet.

Sprinkle the loaf lightly with flour, then dust a wooden spoon handle with flour and press down into the surface of the dough to make a deep cross. This will ensure even cooking… and supposedly lets the fairies out!

Bake for 45–50 minutes, until a golden crust has formed and the bread sounds hollow when tapped on its underside, checking halfway through cooking. If it is already golden at this point, cover loosely with foil for the rest of the cooking time.

Once cooked, transfer the loaf to a wire rack, cover with a clean, damp tea towel and leave to cool. Eat soon after baking, or enjoy toasted for up to 2 days. This loaf also freezes well.

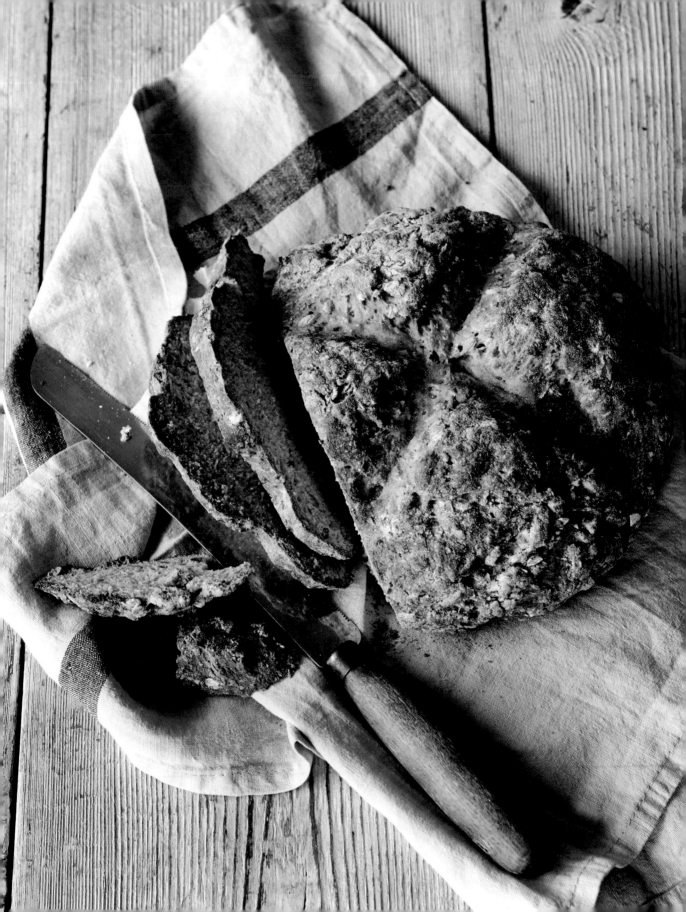

Blueberry buckwheat pancakes

Serves 4

200g buckwheat flour

1 tsp baking powder

¼ tsp ground cinnamon

1 large egg, beaten

250–300ml semi-skimmed milk
or almond milk

150g blueberries

1 tbsp butter

Buckwheat flour is a fantastic, gluten-free alternative to regular flour and these deliciously simple, fruity pancakes make great use of this light, distinctive flour.

Sift the flour, baking powder and cinnamon into a mixing bowl and make a well in the centre.

Add the beaten egg and gradually stir in 250ml of the milk to make a fairly thick, smooth batter, adding more milk if necessary. Stir in the blueberries.

Heat a non-stick frying pan over a medium heat. Use a wad of kitchen paper to wipe the pan with a little butter to grease it. Now add 3 or 4 separate heaped tablespoonfuls of batter to the pan. Once bubbles appear on the surface of each pancake and the top is set at the edges, flip over and fry for a minute or so, until the pancakes are golden and the blueberries are juicy.

Keep warm and repeat with the remaining batter, to make about 12 pancakes in total. Serve alone or with a little maple syrup.

5 WAYS WITH *smoothies*

A healthy, easy-to-digest meal in a glass is that much more appealing than a typical breakfast when your appetite is compromised. Packed with vitamins and minerals to help boost your immune system, smoothies are particularly good following treatment with chemotherapy, when you may be more susceptible to infections. Each of these serves 2.

Banana, ginger, yogurt and lemon
Blend 1 large banana with a chopped 2cm piece of peeled fresh ginger, 50g natural yogurt, 1 tbsp honey, 300ml skimmed milk and the juice of ½ lemon. Pour into glasses.

Avocado, blueberries, spinach and banana
Put ½ peeled avocado, 100g blueberries, a large handful of spinach, 1 banana and the juice of ½ lemon into a blender with 4 tbsp water and blitz until smooth. Serve over ice.

Raspberry, apple and watercress
Put 200g raspberries, 1 peeled, halved and cored apple and a handful of watercress sprigs in a blender with 4 tbsp cold water and blitz until smooth. Pour into glasses over ice cubes.

Beetroot, strawberry and orange
Juice 1 large raw beetroot in an electric juicer, or use 150ml beetroot juice from a carton. Blend the beetroot juice with 100g hulled strawberries and the juice of 2 oranges. Serve chilled.

Pineapple, mint and coconut milk
Blend 300g peeled and cored pineapple flesh, 2 tbsp mint leaves, 150ml coconut milk and 500ml cold water. Pour into glasses over ice cubes.

Soups

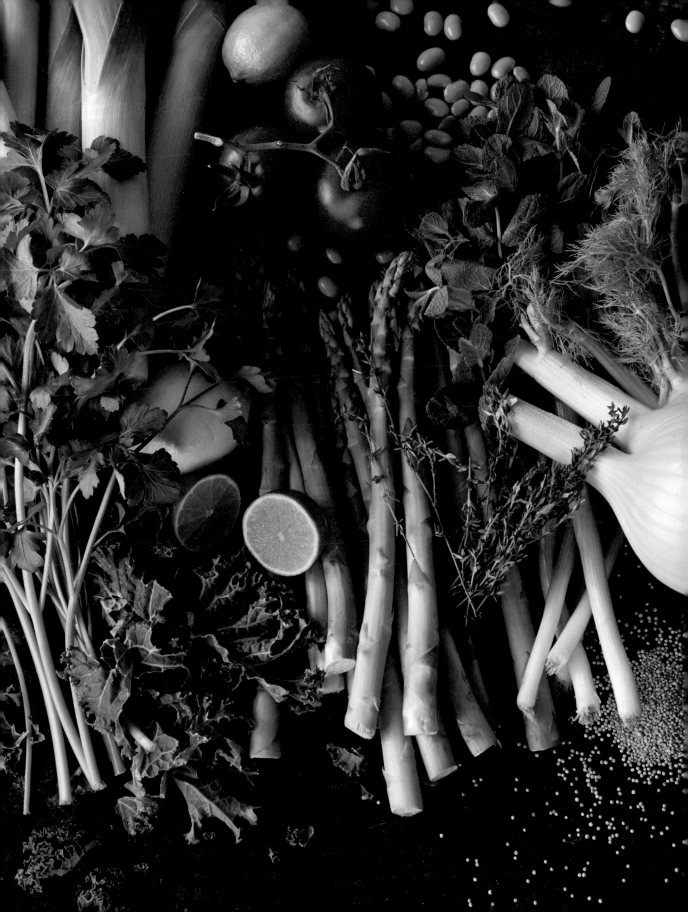

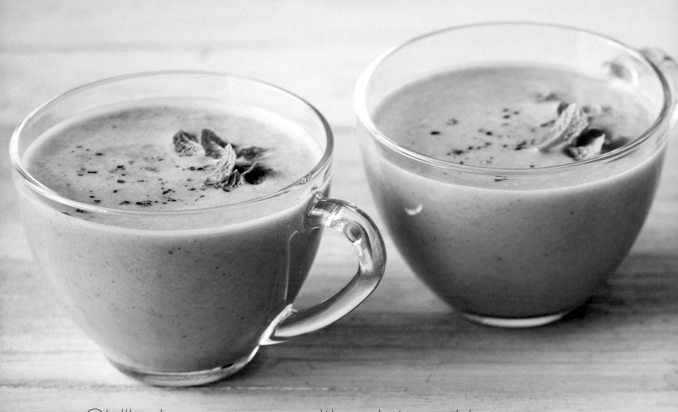

Chilled pea soup with mint and lemon

Serves 4

2 tsp olive oil

1 large shallot, peeled and roughly chopped

4 spring onions, roughly sliced

2 garlic cloves, peeled and crushed

1 litre low-salt vegetable stock

500g podded fresh or frozen peas

A handful of mint leaves, plus extra to garnish

Finely grated zest and juice of ½ lemon

Freshly ground black pepper

A vibrant, refreshing summery soup that is effortless to prepare. Serve it as a starter, or with crusty bread for a light lunch on a hot day.

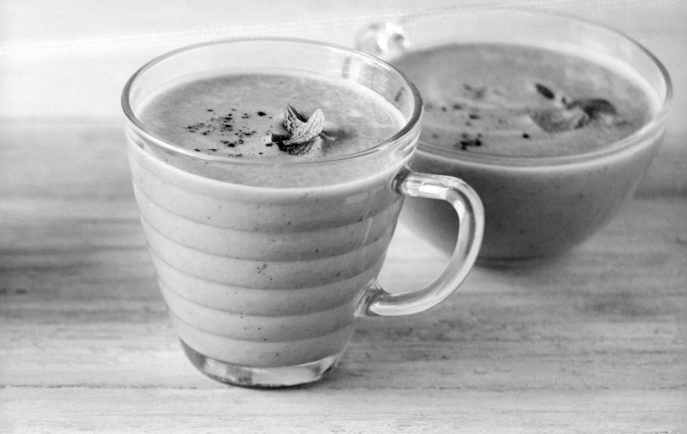

Heat the olive oil in a large saucepan over a medium-low heat. When the oil is hot, add the shallot, spring onions and garlic and fry for 2–3 minutes, until beginning to soften.

Pour in the stock and bring to the boil, then lower the heat and simmer for 5–6 minutes to soften the shallot and spring onions further. Add the peas and mint and cook for another minute, then remove from the heat.

Stir in the lemon zest and juice, then blitz the soup using a blender until smooth.

Pour the soup into a bowl and place over a larger bowl of iced water. Add a couple of lumps of ice to the soup and stir until chilled. Serve seasoned with pepper and garnished with mint.

Asian miso broth with mushrooms

Serves 4

1.2 litres low-salt vegetable stock

2 garlic cloves, peeled and crushed

1cm piece of fresh ginger, peeled and finely grated

4 tbsp white miso paste

125g enoki or shiitake mushrooms, sliced if necessary

100g spring greens, roughly sliced

100g sugar snap peas, sliced in half

A small handful of coriander leaves, to serve

This light and soothing soup is ideal when you might be feeling under the weather. A generous pinch of dried chilli flakes would be a welcome addition if you want to add an extra kick.

Pour the stock into a large saucepan, add the garlic and ginger and bring to a simmer over a medium heat. Simmer gently for 10 minutes to infuse the flavourings.

Stir in the miso, mushrooms, spring greens and sugar snaps. Simmer for 2 minutes and then serve, scattered with coriander.

Ginger, not just a culinary spice

Links between the *Zingiberaceae* (or botanical ginger family) and medicinal health benefits are renowned. Digestive soothing and anti-nausea are typically cited as the primary advantages linked to consuming ginger but its benefits extend beyond this. Cancer patients often describe feverish symptoms for example, and ginger can help alleviate the problem.

Butternut squash and peanut soup

Serves 4–6

1.2 litres low-salt vegetable stock

80g raw, unsalted peanuts
or cashews

1 butternut squash (about 1kg)

2 tsp low-salt soy sauce

3 spring onions, finely sliced

A small handful of coriander
leaves, roughly chopped

Lime wedges, to serve

Based on a simple Vietnamese home-style recipe, this comforting soup is smooth, creamy and nutty, with a nod to the delicious complexity of Asian flavours. An unusual combination, it is sure to become a favourite.

Bring the stock to the boil in a large saucepan over a medium heat. Add the peanuts or cashews and boil for 15 minutes. In the meantime, peel the squash, cut in half, scoop out the seeds and chop into large chunks.

Add the squash to the pan and simmer for a further 12–15 minutes, until both the peanuts and squash are tender. Remove from the heat and blitz in a free-standing blender or with a stick blender until smooth and creamy. Season with the soy sauce.

Serve the soup sprinkled with the sliced spring onions and coriander, with lime wedges on the side for squeezing.

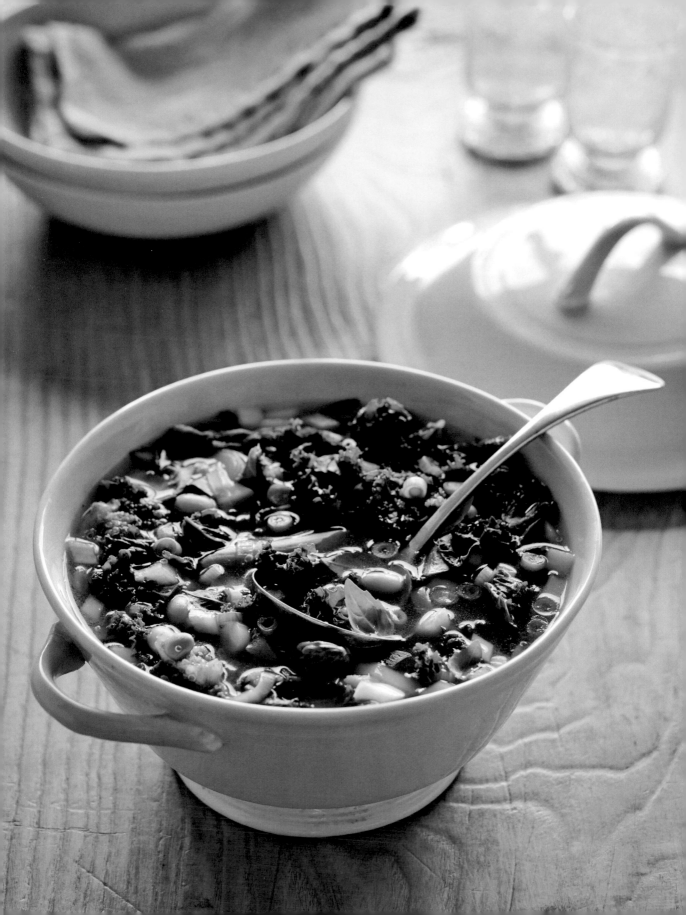

Spring vegetable soup with quinoa

Serves 4

2 tsp olive oil

2 leeks, trimmed, well washed and finely sliced

60g quinoa

1 litre hot, low-salt vegetable stock

1 courgette, diced

100g asparagus spears

100g frozen edamame beans

100g kale, roughly shredded

A handful of basil leaves, roughly chopped

4 spring onions, finely sliced

A squeeze of lemon juice

Quinoa may seem like an unusual addition to soup but it makes for a wholesome and nourishing alternative to pasta or potatoes. This soup is refreshingly light but hearty enough to make for a satisfying meal.

Heat the olive oil in a large saucepan over a medium-low heat. When hot, add the leeks and cook, stirring occasionally, for 5 minutes or until softened, adding a little water if necessary if they look a little dry.

Add the quinoa and pour the stock into the pan. Bring to the boil, then lower the heat and simmer for 5 minutes. Stir in the courgette and continue to cook for another 5 minutes.

Meanwhile, snap off the woody ends of the asparagus and cut the spears into 2cm lengths. Add to the soup with the edamame beans and kale and simmer for another 2 minutes, then remove from the heat.

Serve the soup sprinkled with the chopped basil, sliced spring onions and a squeeze of lemon.

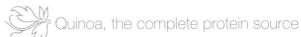 Quinoa, the complete protein source

Proteins are vital for healthy cell functions so they are particularly important if you are undergoing cancer treatment. Quinoa (pronounced *keen-wa*) is an exceptionally good plant source of protein. Unlike other protein-rich grains and legumes, it contains all nine essential amino acids needed by the body. Originating in Latin America, this ancient grain was a staple food of the Incas. Naturally high in fibre and a gluten-free plant source, quinoa is just as valuable to us today.

Spiced red lentil and tomato soup

Serves 4

2 tsp olive oil

1 small red onion, peeled and finely chopped

2 garlic cloves, peeled and crushed

2 tsp ground cumin

1 tsp smoked paprika

1 tsp ground turmeric

120g red split lentils

1 litre low-salt vegetable stock

400g large tomatoes, roughly chopped

A small handful of coriander leaves, roughly chopped

Lemon wedges, to serve

Lightly spiced and bolstered by hearty red lentils and fresh tomatoes, this soup makes for an equally satisfying lunch or supper.

Heat the olive oil in a large saucepan over a medium-low heat. When hot, add the onion and fry gently for 5 minutes until softened, adding a tablespoonful or so of water if it starts to look a little dry.

Add the garlic, cumin, paprika and turmeric and fry for a further minute to roast the spices. Stir in the lentils, stock and chopped tomatoes and bring to the boil, then lower the heat and simmer for 15–20 minutes until the lentils have softened.

Serve just as it is, or if you fancy a smooth soup, whiz in a free-standing blender or using a stick blender until smooth.

Serve sprinkled with coriander, and with lemon wedges on the side for squeezing.

Spices, a cautionary word

Tastebuds are often dulled by cancer treatments and spices can make your food taste more interesting. However, if you experience mouth soreness or ulcers as a consequence of radiation or chemotherapy treatment, you will need to be judicious with spices. For example, capsaicin, found in chilli peppers, is likely to aggravate these conditions. Be reactive to how your body accepts spices in foods, and omit them if necessary. You can always pep up flavour with additional herbs and aromatic vegetables.

Parsnip, apple and ginger soup

Serves 4

2 tsp olive oil

1 small onion, peeled and finely chopped

2.5cm piece of fresh ginger, peeled and finely grated

1 tsp ground cumin

1 tsp ground turmeric

500g parsnips (ideally young and small), peeled and roughly chopped

1 medium-large Bramley apple (about 200g), peeled, cored and roughly chopped

1 litre low-salt vegetable stock

Freshly ground black pepper

Earthy parsnips and sharp-sweet Bramley apples are warmed with ginger and delicate spice in this satisfying soup – perfect to have on standby for a bitingly cold day.

Heat the olive oil in a medium saucepan over a medium-low heat. When hot, add the onion and ginger and fry gently for 5 minutes until softened, adding a little splash of water if the mixture appears a little dry.

Sprinkle the cumin and turmeric into the pan and fry for a minute to roast the spices and release their aromas.

Add the parsnips and apple, give everything a good stir and pour over the stock. Bring to the boil, then lower the heat and simmer for 20 minutes, until the parsnips and apple are very tender.

Blitz the soup in a free-standing blender or using a stick blender until smooth and creamy.

Reheat the soup before serving if necessary, sprinkled lightly with black pepper.

Celeriac soup
with rocket and parsley gremolata

Serves 4

2 tsp olive oil

1 onion, peeled and roughly chopped

2 celery sticks, roughly sliced

1 medium celeriac, peeled and roughly chopped

1.2 litres low-salt vegetable stock

Freshly ground black pepper

For the gremolata

1 garlic clove

Finely grated zest and juice of ½ lemon

A handful of parsley leaves

A handful of rocket

3 tsp extra virgin olive oil

Sweet and earthy, celeriac makes a lovely, satisfying soup. This one is given a refreshing, zesty kick with a splash of gremolata.

Heat the olive oil in a large saucepan over a medium-low heat. When hot, add the onion and celery. Fry gently for about 5 minutes until softened, adding a little water if the veg look a little dry.

Stir in the celeriac and stock and simmer for 20 minutes, until the celeriac is completely soft.

In the meantime, put all of the gremolata ingredients into a food processor and pulse until finely chopped. Add a little water (up to 1 tbsp) to let down the consistency of the gremolata, if preferred.

Using a free-standing or stick blender, blitz the soup until smooth and creamy. Serve topped with a dollop of gremolata and a sprinkling of pepper.

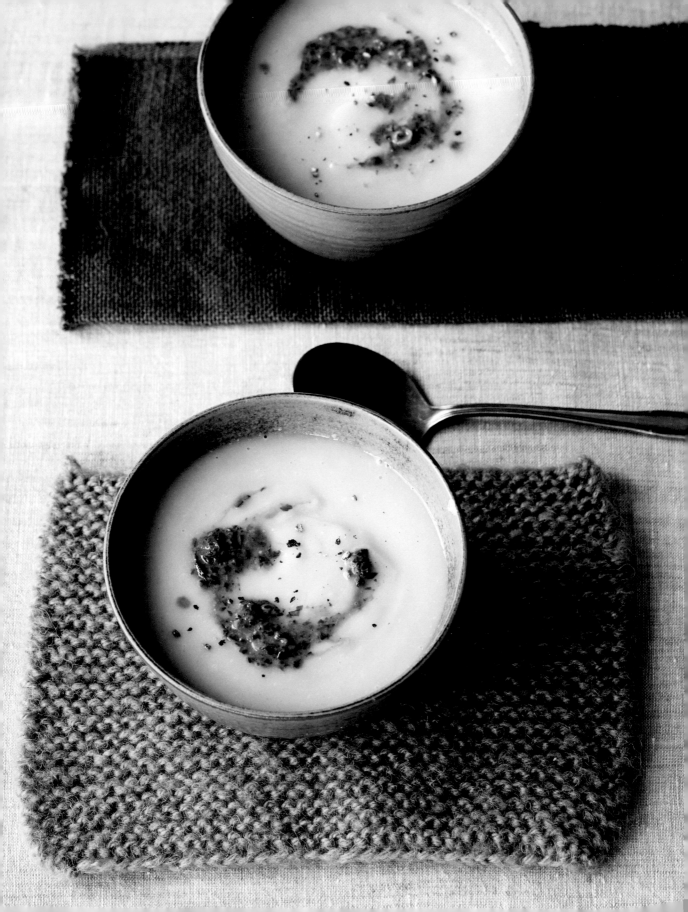

Roasted cauliflower and garlic soup

Serves 4

1 large cauliflower (about 900g), cut into florets

6 garlic cloves (unpeeled)

1 large onion, peeled and roughly sliced

1 tsp caraway seeds

1 tsp thyme leaves

2 tsp olive oil

1.2 litres low-salt vegetable stock

Finely grated zest of ½ lemon

Freshly ground black pepper

Roasting cauliflower brings out the sweet nuttiness of this humble vegetable to delicious effect. Here florets of cauliflower are roasted with garlic cloves, then blitzed with stock to make a wonderful velvety soup with a real depth of flavour.

Preheat the oven to 200°C/Gas 6.

Tip the cauliflower florets into a large bowl and add the garlic and onion. Sprinkle with the caraway seeds and thyme leaves, trickle over the olive oil and toss well to coat the florets.

Spread the cauliflower out on a large baking tray in one layer (you may need to use 2 trays). Roast in the oven for 20–25 minutes, turning halfway through, until the vegetables are lightly burnished and tender.

Take out the garlic cloves and peel away the skins when they are cool enough to handle. Tip the roasted veg mix into a blender, add the peeled garlic cloves and stock and blend until smooth.

Serve topped with a grating of lemon zest and a sprinkling of black pepper.

Jerusalem artichoke and chestnut soup

Serves 4

750g Jerusalem artichokes

Juice of ½ lemon

2 tsp sunflower oil

1 onion, peeled and finely chopped

2 garlic cloves, peeled and crushed

1 tbsp thyme leaves, roughly chopped

100g vacuum-packed peeled chestnuts

1 litre low-salt chicken or vegetable stock

Freshly ground black pepper

A small handful of parsley leaves, roughly chopped, to serve

This wonderfully warming soup is a great one to make over the Christmas holiday – it's an ideal starter to precede a traditional Boxing Day cold spread.

Peel and roughly chop the artichokes, immediately immersing them in a bowl of cold water with the lemon juice added to prevent discoloration.

Heat the oil in a large saucepan over a medium-low heat. When hot, add the onion and fry gently for about 5 minutes until softened, adding a little water if necessary, if it looks a little dry. Add the garlic and thyme and fry for a further minute.

Drain the artichokes and add them to the pan along with the chestnuts. Give the mixture a good stir and pour in the stock. Bring to the boil, then lower the heat slightly and simmer for 10–15 minutes until the artichokes are tender.

Blitz the mixture in a blender until smooth, season with black pepper and sprinkle with chopped parsley to serve.

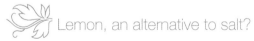 Lemon, an alternative to salt?

A squeeze of lemon can alter the flavour profile of any dish, sweet or savoury. Acidity – like saltiness – in our mouths acts as a stimulant for salivation, increasing our desire for a food. Take on board health concerns about the amount of salt we consume and add a squeeze of lemon as you serve food, instead of reaching for the salt mill. Of course, if you are undergoing chemotherapy and experiencing mouth soreness as a consequence, seasoning with lemon juice isn't advisable as it can aggravate the problem.

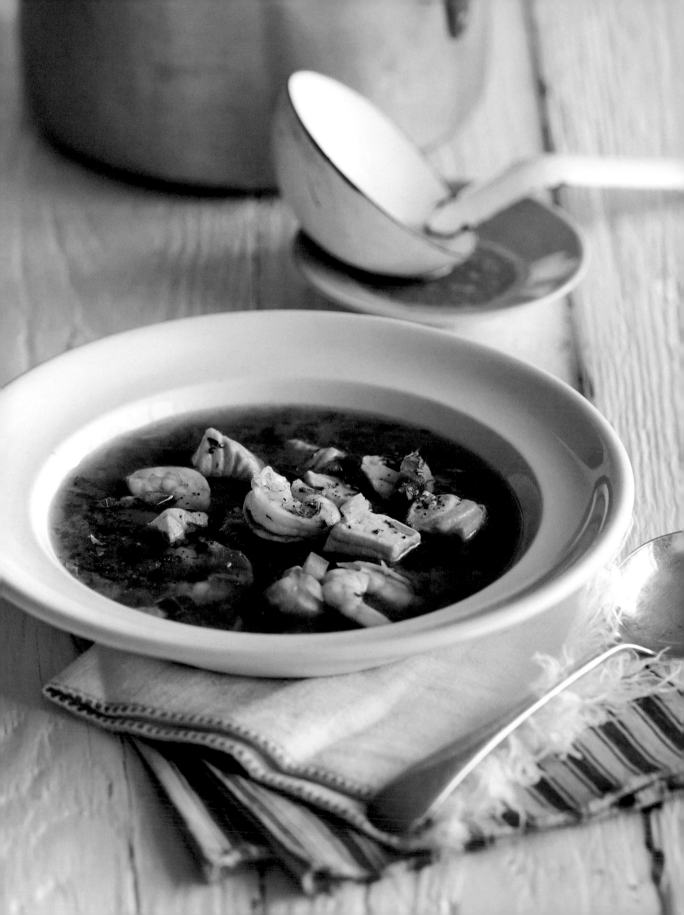

Seafood soup
with saffron and fennel

Serves 4

2 tsp olive oil

2 shallots, peeled and finely
chopped or sliced

1 inner celery stalk, finely
chopped

1 small fennel bulb, finely
chopped

2 garlic cloves, peeled and
crushed

A pinch of saffron strands

1 litre low-salt fish stock

2 thyme sprigs, leaves picked

2 large tomatoes, quartered,
deseeded and finely diced

250g skinless salmon fillets,
cut into 2cm pieces

180g raw tiger prawns, deveined

A small handful of parsley leaves,
chopped

Saffron, fennel and seafood are made for each other.
In this delicious Mediterranean-style soup, the fragrant
subtlety of saffron brings out the delicate aroma of
fennel and the sweetness of the salmon and prawns.

Heat the olive oil in a large saucepan over a medium-low heat.
When hot, add the shallots, celery and fennel and fry gently,
stirring occasionally, for 8–10 minutes until softened, adding a little
water if the mixture seems a little dry.

Add the garlic and fry for a further minute, then crumble the saffron
between your fingers and sprinkle directly into the pan. Pour in the
stock, stir in the thyme and tomatoes and bring to the boil.

Add the salmon pieces to the pan, lower the heat and simmer for
2 minutes, then stir in the prawns and simmer for another minute
or two, until they are opaque and pink.

Serve the soup scattered with chopped parsley.

Vietnamese chicken soup (pho ga)

Serves 4–6

For the broth

2 onions, peeled and halved

4cm piece of fresh ginger, peeled and roughly sliced

2 cinnamon sticks

1 tsp black peppercorns

3 star anise

1 oven-ready medium chicken (about 1.5kg)

1 carrot, peeled and roughly chopped

2 celery sticks, roughly chopped

1.5 litres good quality, low-salt chicken stock (preferably fresh)

To assemble the soup

1 Chinese cabbage, shredded

1 tbsp fish sauce

2 tsp maple syrup

6 spring onions, sliced

100g beansprouts

A handful each of mint, coriander and basil leaves

1 red chilli, sliced (optional)

To serve

Lime wedges

Fragrant, soothing and easy on the stomach, this aromatic chicken soup is a great recipe to have in your repertoire and leaves you some leftover chicken for a salad or sandwiches.

Preheat the grill to high. Lay the onions and ginger out on a grill tray and grill for 4–5 minutes, turning occasionally, until tinged with brown.

Transfer the onion and ginger to a large stockpot or flameproof casserole dish (large enough to hold a whole chicken) and add the cinnamon, peppercorns and star anise.

Place the chicken in the pot and tuck the carrot and celery around it. Pour over the stock and top up with enough water to just cover the chicken. Place over a medium heat and bring to the boil.

Turn the heat down slightly and simmer very gently for 50 minutes to 1 hour, or until the chicken is completely cooked through and tender. Remove the chicken from the pot and set aside to cool slightly. Reduce the stock down by boiling if necessary until you have 1.2 litres. Strain.

Peel off and discard the skin from the chicken, then remove the meat from the bone and shred into bite-sized pieces.

Return the stock to the heat and add the Chinese cabbage, fish sauce and maple syrup. Simmer for 1 minute.

Ladle the soup into warm bowls, add a portion of chicken meat to each bowl, then scatter over the spring onions, beansprouts, herbs and chilli, if using. Serve with lime wedges for squeezing.

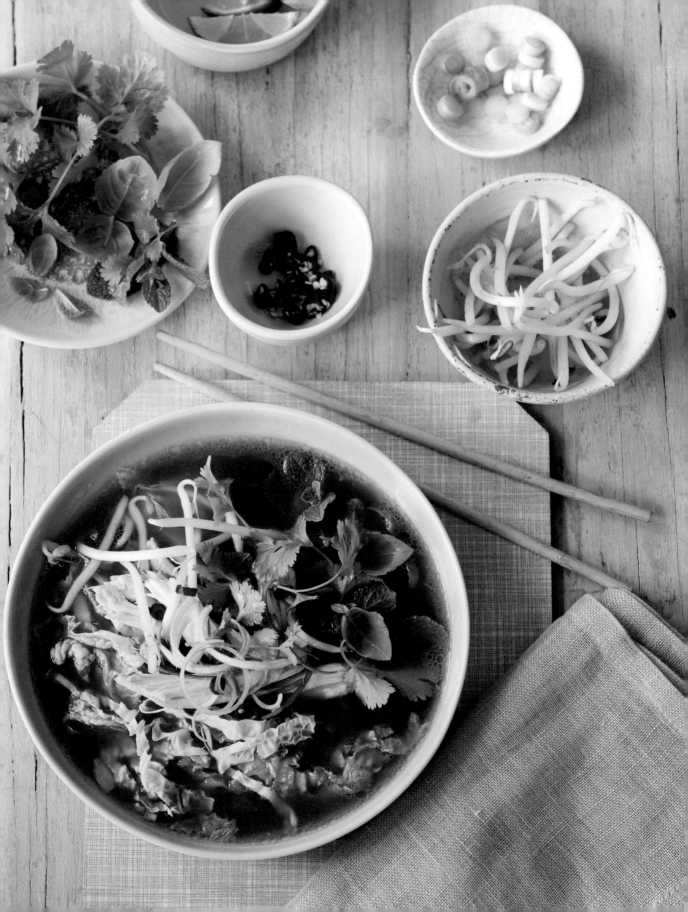

Italian bean soup
with basil and parsley pesto

Serves 4

2 tsp olive oil

1 onion, peeled and finely
chopped

1 carrot, peeled and finely
chopped

3 garlic cloves, peeled
and crushed

2 bay leaves

2 thyme sprigs

1 tbsp tomato purée

1 courgette, diced

1 litre low-salt vegetable stock

400g tomatoes, quartered,
deseeded and roughly chopped

400g can cannellini beans

200g Savoy cabbage, shredded

For the pesto

1 garlic clove, peeled

A handful each of basil and
parsley leaves

20g Parmesan, finely grated

2 tsp olive oil

4 tbsp water

This hearty vegetable and bean soup, served topped with a dollop of easy homemade pesto, is wonderfully warming and sustaining for a chilly wintry day.

Heat the olive oil in a large saucepan over a medium-low heat. When hot, add the onion and carrot and fry for about 5 minutes until softened, adding a little water if necessary, to moisten. Add the garlic and fry for another minute.

Now add the bay leaves, thyme, tomato purée, courgette and stock. Bring to a simmer and cook for 10 minutes, then add the tomatoes, beans and cabbage and simmer for another 5 minutes to soften the cabbage.

To make the pesto, simply put the garlic, herbs, Parmesan and olive oil in a food processor and blitz to a thick paste. Drizzle in the cold water to let the pesto down, and pulse briefly.

Serve the soup topped with a dollop of pesto.

5 WAYS WITH *nuts and seeds*

A sprinkling of nuts and seeds adds flavour and texture to meals and snacks, with a plethora of nutritional benefits. In particular, flavonoids (in the skins on almonds) and phytosterols (concentrated in sesame seeds) help to reduce blood cholesterol levels. Why not add a sprinkling to your breakfast, salad or soup…

Hemp, flax and sunflower seed sprinkle
Mix together 4 tbsp each of shelled hemp seeds, flax seeds and sunflower seeds. Stir though 2 tsp ground cinnamon and sprinkle over smoothies, porridge or Bircher muesli (page 23).

Pepper and maple pecans
Toast 100g pecan halves in a frying pan until fragrant, then add ¼ tsp ground black pepper and 2 tsp maple syrup and dry-fry until sticky. Leave to cool and enjoy as a snack, or sprinkle over salads, or chop up and sprinkle over Parsnip, apple and ginger soup (page 49).

Pine nut, oregano and tomato mix
Blitz 8 sun-dried tomatoes (not in oil) with 2 tbsp pine nuts and 2 tsp dried oregano in a food processor until fairly fine. Delicious sprinkled over salads and soups, such as the Italian bean soup opposite.

Soy baked almonds and sesame seeds
Mix together 100g raw almonds, 2 tbsp sesame seeds, 1 tsp vegetable oil and 1 tbsp low-salt soy sauce. Roast in the oven at 180°C/Gas 4 for 10–15 minutes, let cool slightly, then chop roughly. Great as a snack or sprinkled over Asian salads, such as Chicken, cashew and mandarin salad (page 77), for added crunch.

Paprika sunflower seeds
Mix 100g sunflower seeds with 1 tsp olive oil and 1 tsp smoked paprika and toast in a pan for a few minutes. Delicious sprinkled over salads, such as Puy lentil and halloumi salad (page 80).

Salads

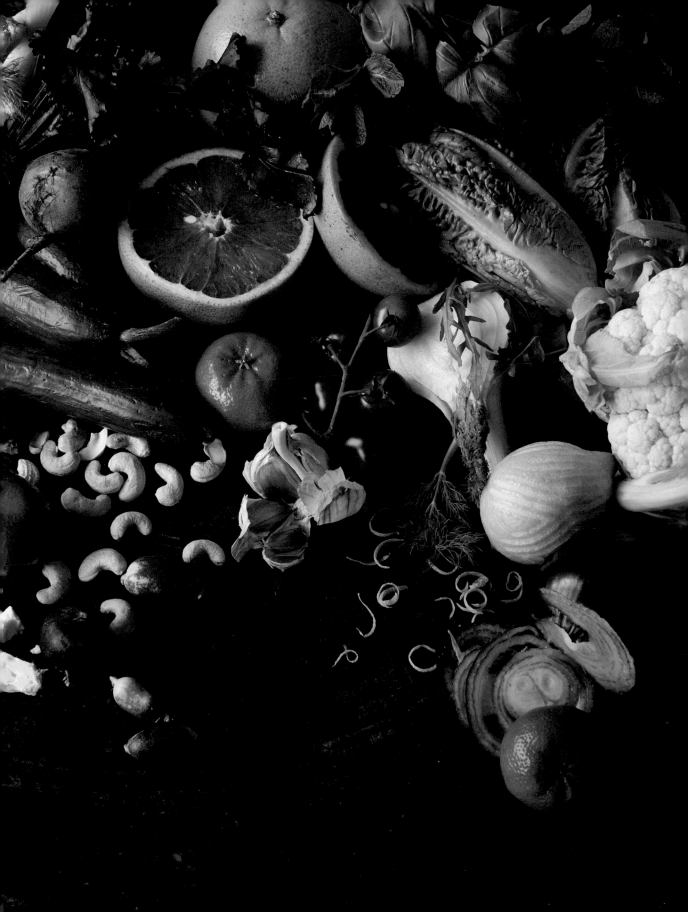

Fennel and citrus salad

Serves 4

2 fennel bulbs, tough outer layer removed

1½ tsp fennel seeds

2 large oranges

1 large pink grapefruit

100g rocket or watercress leaves

Juice of 2 limes

3 tsp olive oil

Freshly ground black pepper

This refreshing, zingy salad, with its contrasting tastes and textures, makes a lovely light lunch served on its own. It also partners oily fish such as mackerel, salmon or trout beautifully.

Slice the fennel very finely, place in a large bowl and sprinkle over the fennel seeds.

To prepare the citrus fruits, cut the top and bottom off the oranges and grapefruit to reveal the flesh and then cut the pith and peel away in vertical strips. Now cut either side of the membranes to release the segments, adding them to the fennel as you go.

Once all the segments have been removed, squeeze out the juice from the orange and grapefruit core and membranes over the bowl of fennel and segments. Set aside for 5 minutes to allow the fennel to soften slightly.

When you are ready to serve the salad, toss through the rocket or watercress. Mix the lime juice and olive oil together and trickle over the salad. Season liberally with pepper and serve.

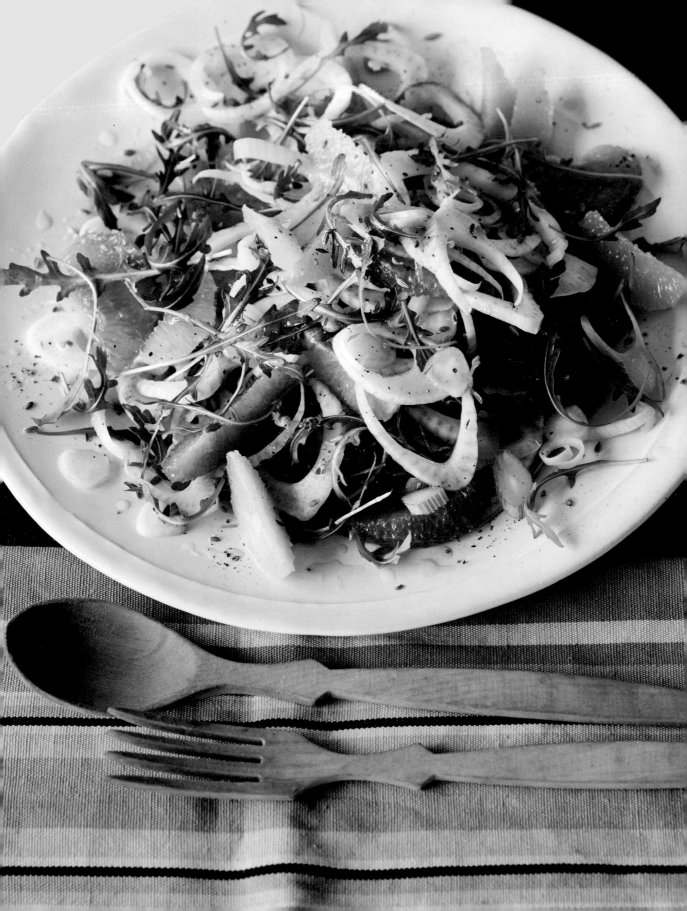

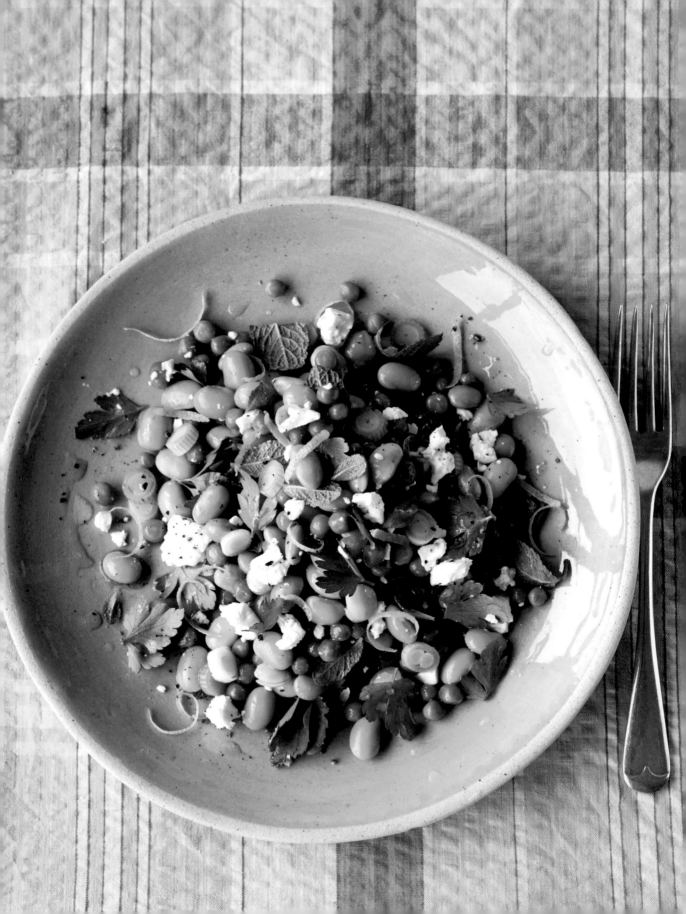

Edamame bean, pea and lemon salad

Serves 4

200g podded fresh or frozen edamame beans

200g podded fresh or frozen peas

Finely pared zest (in strips) and juice of 1 lemon

4 spring onions, finely sliced

A small handful of parsley leaves, roughly chopped

A small handful of mint leaves, roughly chopped

40g light feta or sheep's milk cheese, crumbled

Freshly ground black pepper

Sweet, tender peas and edamame beans marry perfectly with sharp lemon and feta to make a light salad that will go from chopping board to table in minutes.

Bring a medium pan of water to the boil. Add the edamame beans and simmer for 4 minutes. Now add the peas and heat for a further minute, then drain and run under cold water to refresh.

Combine the cooled beans and peas with the remaining ingredients and stir to disperse the flavours. Season with pepper to taste and serve immediately.

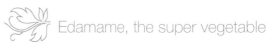 Edamame, the super vegetable

These green soy beans are the only vegetable regarded as a complete protein food – as they contain all nine essential amino acids. Edamame are also a good source of vitamins, minerals, fibre and phytoestrogens, which are thought to inhibit the growth of cancer cells. It is difficult to find fresh edamame but the frozen beans are available all year round. Frozen soon after picking and podding, their nutrient content is well preserved.

Sugar snap pea and quinoa salad with pistachios

Serves 4

200g quinoa

500ml low-salt vegetable stock or water

200g sugar snap peas, halved lengthways

4 spring onions, finely sliced

A small handful each of chives, parsley and mint leaves, roughly chopped

40g raw, unsalted pistachio nuts, roughly chopped

1½ tsp maple syrup

Juice of 1 lemon

1 tbsp olive oil

A pinch of dried chilli flakes (optional)

Crunchy, sweet sugar snaps and pistachios add a vibrancy to mellow quinoa, which can be cooked and stored in the fridge the day before for convenience. Don't be concerned if you haven't got all the herbs to hand – a mix of two will be just as delicious.

To cook the quinoa, bring the stock or water to the boil in a medium pan and add the quinoa. Simmer over a medium heat for 15 minutes, or until the quinoa has absorbed the water and is tender but still has a little bite to it, adding a little more water if necessary.

Tip the quinoa into a sieve and briefly run under cold water to cool, then set aside.

Put the sliced sugar snaps into a salad bowl and scatter over the spring onions, herbs and pistachios.

Whisk together the maple syrup, lemon juice, olive oil and chilli flakes, if using, and pour this dressing over the salad. Add the quinoa, give everything a good mix and serve.

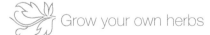 Grow your own herbs

Herbs are a complex resource, rich in antioxidant vitamins and minerals. As they are harvested, however, their nutritional value diminishes. So, grow them at home – in pots on a windowsill or patio – if you do not have a garden – and pick them just before adding to dishes for maximum flavour and nutritional value.

Asparagus and white bean salad

Serves 4

400g asparagus spears

2 tsp olive oil

1 tsp soy sauce

2 shallots, peeled and finely chopped

Juice of 1 lemon

2 x 400g cans cannellini beans, drained

2 large tomatoes, quartered, deseeded and roughly chopped

A handful of parsley leaves, roughly chopped

2 tbsp finely chopped chives

Freshly ground black pepper

Crisp-grilled homegrown asparagus and creamy white beans are brought together with a lemony soy dressing for a delightfully simple late-spring lunch.

Preheat the grill to high.

Snap off the woody ends of the asparagus and cut the spears into roughly 5cm lengths. Toss the prepared asparagus in 1 tsp of the olive oil and season with the soy sauce and black pepper. Transfer to a foil-lined baking tray and grill for 5–6 minutes until tender and tinged with brown but still crisp within. Set aside to cool slightly.

Meanwhile, stir the shallots with the lemon juice and set aside to mellow the acerbic tang of the shallots.

Combine the cannellini beans and tomatoes in a large bowl and add the lemony shallots. Toss to mix and then add the asparagus and chopped herbs. Toss lightly and serve.

Middle Eastern beetroot salad with a grapefruit dressing

Serves 4

Finely pared zest (in strips) and juice of 1 pink grapefruit

2 tsp maple syrup

4 medium beetroot (about 150g each)

½ red onion, peeled and finely sliced

Juice of 1 lemon

100g radishes, sliced or cut into quarters

A small handful each of dill, basil, coriander and parsley leaves

¼ tsp ground sumac

Raw beetroot springs to life in this salad, which is adapted from a traditional Middle Eastern recipe. It takes a little time to prepare but the earthy and zingy sweet result will have you making this salad time and time again.

First, prepare the dressing: put the grapefruit zest and juice and the maple syrup into a saucepan and bring to the boil over a medium heat. Lower the heat and simmer for 5–10 minutes, until of a light, syrupy consistency. Pour into a bowl or jug and set the dressing aside to cool while you prepare the other ingredients.

Peel and very finely slice the beetroot, using a mandoline if you have one.

Tip the sliced beetroot and red onion into a salad bowl and drizzle over the lemon juice. Set aside for 5 minutes so that the lemon juice can soften the beetroot slightly and mellow the acerbic tang of the onion.

Combine the beetroot and onion with the radishes and herbs and sprinkle over the sumac. Drizzle over the dressing and serve.

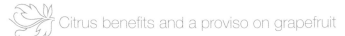 Citrus benefits and a proviso on grapefruit

Citrus fruits are an excellent source of vitamin C, an important antioxidant that helps to boost our immune system. They also contain flavonoids, which may have anti-cancer properties. You should, however, be aware that grapefruit can interfere with the action of certain drugs, including some used to treat breast cancer. Be advised by your doctor or dietitian as to whether you should avoid this fruit if you are undergoing treatment.

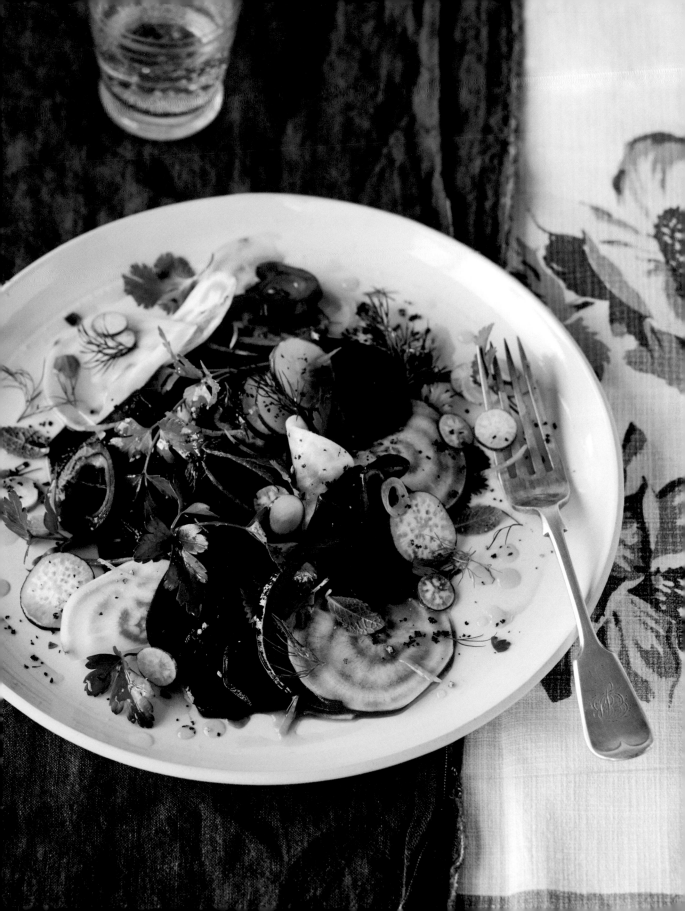

Butternut squash and pearl barley salad

Serves 4

150g pearl barley

500g butternut squash

1 tsp ground cinnamon

1 tbsp plus 2 tsp olive oil

4 spring onions, sliced

A handful of parsley leaves, roughly chopped

40g raw almonds, roughly chopped

40g light feta cheese, crumbled

Juice of 2 lemons

½ tsp ground sumac

Freshly ground black pepper (optional)

This wholesome, delicately spiced autumnal salad can be eaten warm or cold. The feta adds a salty tang but the salad is also delicious without it, so omit it if preferred.

Preheat the oven to 200°C/Gas 6.

Bring a large pan of water to the boil. Rinse the pearl barley in a sieve to remove the excess starch, then add to the boiling water and cook for 30 minutes, until tender but not too soft.

Meanwhile, peel and halve the squash, scoop out the seeds and cut into 1–2cm chunks. Put into a bowl. Sprinkle with the cinnamon and 1 tbsp olive oil and toss until the squash is well coated with spice. Transfer to a large roasting tin and roast for 20–25 minutes, until tinged with brown and tender.

Check the pearl barley and once it is cooked, drain, rinse briefly with cold water and drain thoroughly.

Combine the squash and pearl barley in a large salad bowl and sprinkle over the spring onions, parsley, almonds and feta.

Whisk together the remaining 2 tsp olive oil, lemon juice and sumac and pour over the salad. Toss to combine and finish with a little black pepper, if liked. Either serve straight away, or allow to cool before serving.

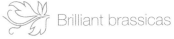 Brilliant brassicas

From a nutritional perspective, brassicas such as kale, broccoli and cauliflower, are impressive. Packed with vital antioxidant vitamins and minerals, a low-calorie source of protein and an excellent source of fibre, they also contain glucosinolates. Research studies have suggested that these phytonutrients can reduce the risk of developing certain cancers.

Roasted cauliflower salad with a tahini dressing

Serves 4

1 medium cauliflower, cut into bite-sized florets

4 garlic cloves (unpeeled)

2 tsp olive oil

1 small red onion, peeled and cut into wedges

1½ tsp ground cumin

1 tsp ground turmeric

Finely grated zest and juice of 1 lemon

2 tbsp tahini

4 tbsp water

80g baby leaf salad

A small handful of parsley leaves, roughly chopped

A small handful of coriander leaves, roughly chopped

Freshly ground black pepper

With its inviting, spicy flavours, this salad is lovely served warm for lunch. Alternatively the cauliflower can be roasted the day before – to allow time for the flavours to mingle – and the salad served cold the following day.

Preheat the oven to 200°C/Gas 6.

Place the cauliflower in a large bowl. Peel and crush two of the garlic cloves and add them to the cauliflower with the olive oil, onion wedges, cumin, turmeric, lemon zest and half the lemon juice. Season with pepper to taste.

Give everything a good stir so the cauliflower is golden with spice and everything is well dispersed, then tip the mixture into a large baking tray or roasting tin and tuck the remaining whole garlic cloves in amongst the vegetables.

Roast in the oven for 20–25 minutes until the cauliflower is tinged with brown and tender but still slightly crisp within, turning the florets halfway through cooking. Set aside to cool slightly, picking out and reserving the whole garlic cloves.

To make the dressing, squeeze the softened roasted garlic out from their skins and mash with a fork. Mix in the tahini, remaining lemon juice and water until smooth.

Toss the salad leaves and herbs together in a large salad bowl, then add the roasted cauliflower mixture. Pour the dressing over the salad. Gently toss everything together to coat in the dressing and serve.

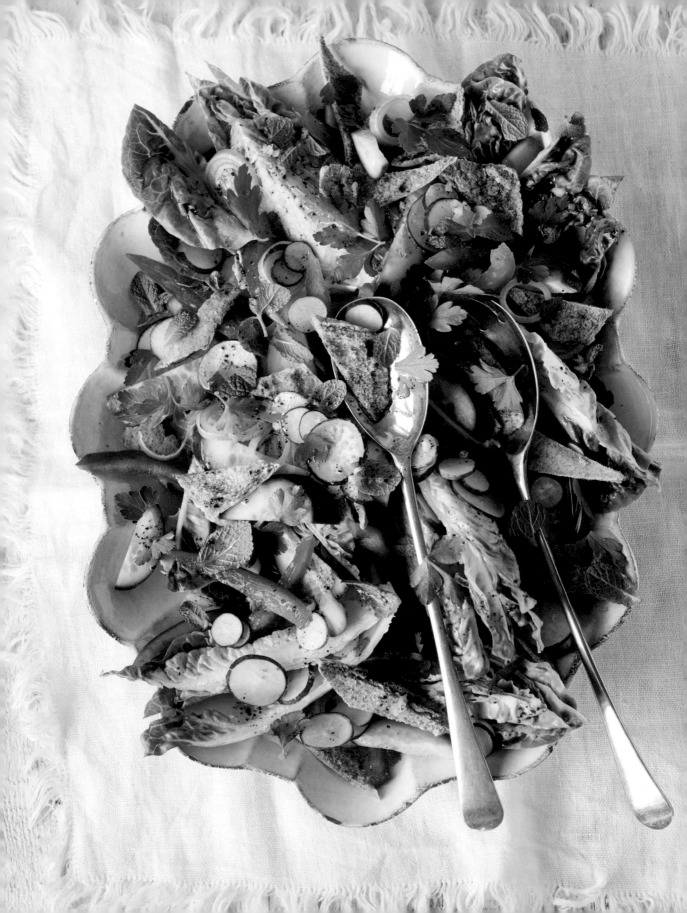

Fattoush salad

Serves 4

½ large cucumber

3 Little Gem lettuces

4 large tomatoes, quartered, deseeded and sliced

8 radishes, sliced

2 small shallots, peeled and finely sliced

A small handful of mint leaves, roughly chopped

A small handful of flat-leaf parsley leaves

2 wholemeal pitta breads

3 tsp olive oil

2 garlic cloves, peeled and crushed

Juice of 1 lemon

1 tsp ground sumac

This fresh Middle Eastern salad is the perfect way to enjoy some of the finest salad ingredients summer offers: tomatoes, radishes, lettuce, cucumber and herbs. Tossed in a lemon, garlic and sumac dressing with toasted pitta it's an irresistible combination.

Preheat the grill to medium.

Halve the cucumber lengthways, slice and place in a large salad bowl. Separate the lettuce leaves, tearing larger leaves in half, and add to the bowl. Add the tomatoes, radishes, shallots and herbs and toss together.

Put the pitta breads into a separate bowl. Whisk together the olive oil and garlic. Drizzle half of this mixture over the pittas and turn the pittas to coat well. Lay on a non-stick baking tray and grill for 2–3 minutes until lightly toasted and golden, turning as necessary. Cut into bite-sized pieces and set aside.

Whisk the lemon juice and sumac into the remaining oil and garlic mixture and trickle over the salad. Add the toasted pitta, toss to mix and serve.

Watermelon Greek salad

Serves 4

600g ripe watermelon

1 cucumber

2 large tomatoes, quartered, deseeded and sliced

½ small red onion, peeled and finely sliced

8 black olives, pitted and quartered

2 tsp olive oil

Juice of 1 lemon

1 tsp dried oregano

A small handful of mint leaves, roughly chopped if large

80g light feta cheese, crumbled

Naturally sweet, watermelon is a lovely, colourful addition to a classic Greek salad. A breeze to prepare, this wonderfully refreshing salad is just the thing to enjoy for lunch on a hot summer's day.

Cut the watermelon into bite-sized chunks, slicing away the thick rind, and place on a large platter.

Halve the cucumber lengthways and scoop out the seeds, then slice roughly. Add the cucumber to the watermelon with the tomatoes, red onion and black olives.

Mix together the olive oil and lemon juice and trickle over the salad, then scatter over the oregano, mint and feta. Give everything a good stir before serving.

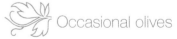 Occasional olives

Olives and olive oil are an integral part of the Mediterranean diet, which is associated with lower incidences of heart disease and cancer. The mono-unsaturated nature of their fat content does, indeed, give them a healthy profile and they also contain antioxidants and minerals. However, the olives we consume have been cured in salt or brine and are therefore high in sodium. So, while they have a role to play in adding flavour to salads and other dishes, both black and green olives should be consumed in moderation.

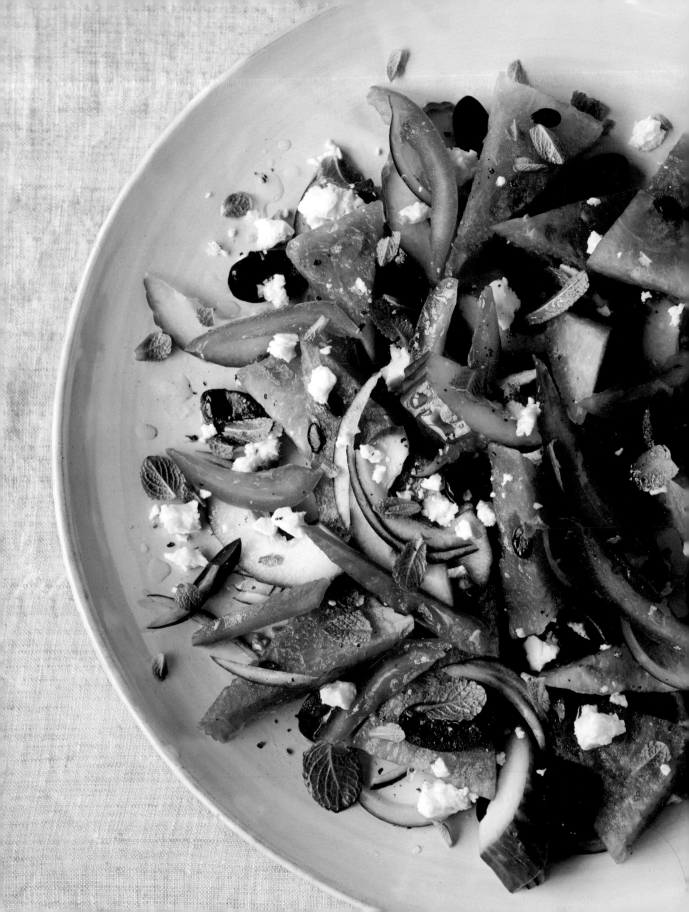

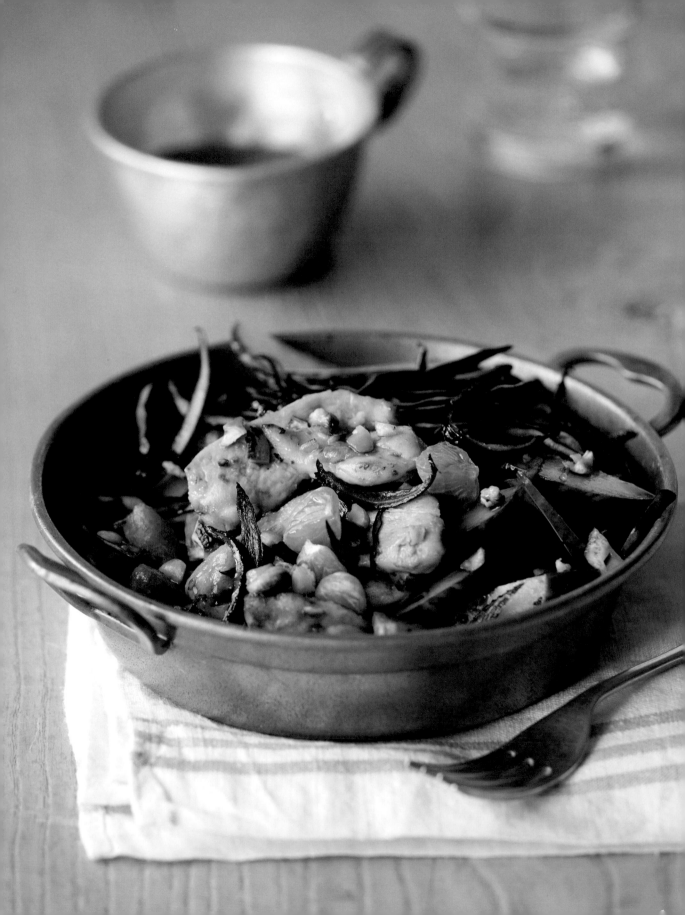

Chicken, cashew and mandarin salad

Serves 4

560g skinless, boneless chicken breast

2 tsp olive oil

2 garlic cloves, peeled and crushed

2cm piece of fresh ginger, peeled and grated

½ red onion, peeled and sliced

40g cashew nuts, very roughly chopped

2 mandarins or clementines

1 cucumber, halved lengthways and sliced

½ small red cabbage, finely sliced

A small handful of coriander leaves, roughly chopped

2 tsp low-salt soy sauce

Juice of 2 limes

This Asian-inspired salad is enticingly bright and flavoursome. It is delicious served warm or cold, as a satisfying lunch or supper.

Preheat the grill to medium-high. Cut the chicken into strips, about 1cm thick, and place in a bowl. Add the olive oil, garlic, ginger, red onion and cashew nuts and toss to mix. Set aside whilst the grill heats up.

Transfer the chicken mixture to a foil-lined baking tray and place under the grill. Grill for 3 minutes, then turn the chicken pieces, onion and cashews over and grill for a further 3 minutes, or until the chicken is just cooked through. Remove from the grill and leave to cool slightly.

In the meantime, finely grate the zest from the mandarins and set aside. Peel the fruit and roughly chop the flesh.

Put the mandarin pieces in a large bowl with the grated zest, cucumber, cabbage and coriander and toss together. Stir through the chicken, cashews and onion.

Whisk together the soy sauce and lime juice to make a dressing. Trickle over the salad and serve.

Thai beef salad

Serves 4

560g rump steak, 2cm thick (about 2 steaks), trimmed of any outer fat

1 tsp vegetable oil

1 cucumber

200g cherry tomatoes, quartered

A small handful each of basil, mint and coriander leaves, roughly chopped

4 spring onions, finely sliced

A handful of ready-to-eat beansprouts and/or sprouting seeds

2 tsp fish sauce

2 tsp maple syrup

1½ tbsp lime juice

1 red chilli, deseeded and finely chopped (optional)

This aromatic and spicy salad is typically laced with sugar but this lighter version uses a little healthier maple syrup instead to complete the authentic combination of sweet, salty and sour flavours.

Remove the steaks from the fridge 15 minutes before cooking. Place a non-stick frying pan over a medium-high heat. Pat the steaks dry with kitchen paper.

Add the oil to the hot pan and when it is really hot, add the steaks. Cook for 1½ minutes each side for rare, 2 minutes each side for medium and 2¼ minutes each side for well done, turning once only. Remove from the pan and set aside to rest while you prepare the salad.

Halve the cucumber lengthways and cut across into slices. Place in a large salad bowl with the tomatoes, herbs, spring onions and sprouts. Toss to combine.

Stir together the fish sauce, maple syrup, lime juice and chilli, if using, to make the dressing.

Finely slice the steak, combine with the salad ingredients and pour over the dressing. Let stand for a few minutes to allow the dressing to soak into the steak, then serve.

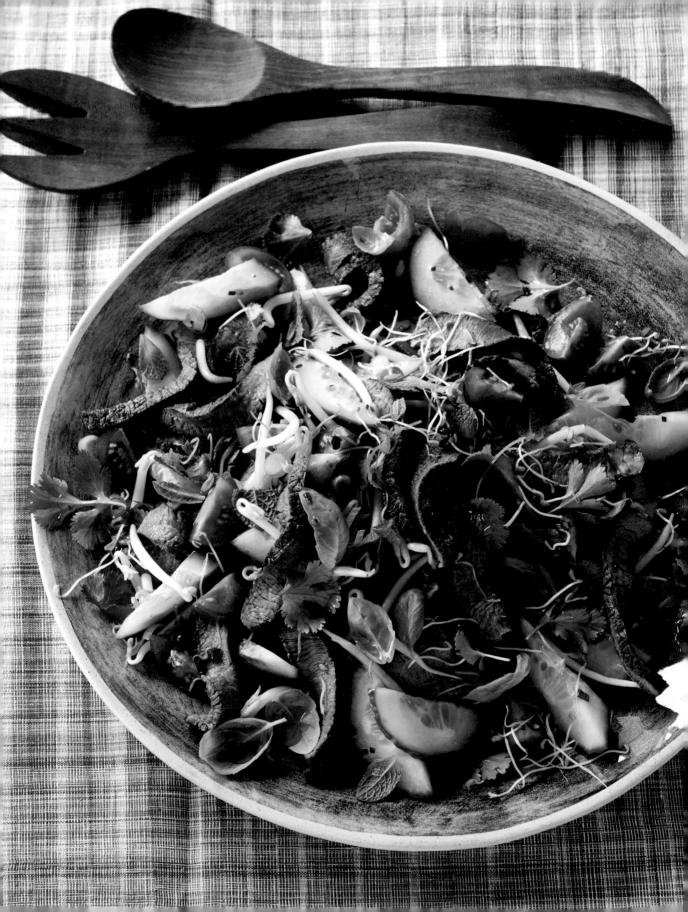

Puy lentil and halloumi salad with lemon and garlic

Serves 4

200g Puy lentils, rinsed

½ red onion, peeled and finely chopped

Finely grated zest and juice of ½ lemon

1 tsp sunflower oil

2 garlic cloves, peeled and crushed

120g light halloumi, cut into 8 slices

200g cherry or baby plum tomatoes, halved

80g rocket leaves

A handful of parsley leaves, roughly chopped

2 tsp balsamic vinegar

Freshly ground black pepper

Wonderfully savoury, halloumi is lovely fried with fragrant lemon zest and garlic and works beautifully with wholesome lentils and sweet tomatoes.

To cook the lentils, bring a large pan of water to the boil, add the lentils and simmer for 20–25 minutes, until tender but not too soft.

Meanwhile, put the onion into a small bowl, add the lemon juice and set aside while you prepare the remaining ingredients.

Mix together the oil, garlic, lemon zest and halloumi. Place a large non-stick frying pan over a medium heat. When hot, add the halloumi and fry for 1–2 minutes on each side until a golden crust has formed, then remove from the heat.

Drain the lentils as soon as they are cooked. While still warm, toss them with the tomatoes, rocket, parsley and balsamic vinegar. Season with pepper to taste.

Divide the salad between 4 plates. Top each serving with 2 slices of grilled halloumi and serve warm.

5 WAYS WITH *tomatoes*

'A tomato a day keeps inflammation at bay.' Lycopene – a potentially powerful carotenoid found in tomatoes – is widely believed to reduce inflammation, which contributes to the development of cancer and several other diseases. Try these lovely, simple ideas for fresh tomatoes.

Slow-roasted tomatoes with garlic and thyme

Place 400g halved cherry tomatoes on a baking tray and sprinkle with 4 crushed garlic cloves, 4 tsp thyme leaves, 2 tbsp olive oil and a grinding of black pepper. Roast in the oven at 140°C/Gas 1 for 1¼ hours. Set aside to cool. 4–6 servings

Fresh tomato and herb dressing

In a blender or food processor, whiz 300g cherry tomatoes with 6 spring onions, 2 roughly chopped garlic cloves, 4 tsp olive oil, the juice of 2 lemons, a good pinch of paprika and 2 tbsp roughly chopped herbs (chervil, parsley or mint) until smooth. Use to dress your favourite salad. 6–8 servings

Grilled cherry tomatoes with balsamic vinegar and garlic

Lay 400g cherry tomatoes on a baking tray. Mix together 4 crushed garlic cloves, 1 tsp dried oregano, 2 tsp clear honey, 4 tsp balsamic vinegar and 4 tsp olive oil and drizzle over the tomatoes. Grill under a high heat for 6–8 minutes until tinged with brown. Delicious with grilled steak, tuna or aubergines. 4 servings

Gazpacho salad

Deseed and roughly chop 6 large tomatoes and mix with 1 finely chopped red onion, 2 roughly chopped, cored and deseeded red peppers, 1 roughly chopped cucumber, 4 roughly sliced Little Gem lettuces and a large handful of roughly chopped parsley. Mix together 2 tbsp olive oil and 4 tsp red wine vinegar and drizzle over the salad. Serve with chunks of wholemeal bread. 4–6 servings

Quick tomato salsa

Finely chop 8 large tomatoes and mix with 1 finely chopped red onion, 2 crushed garlic cloves, the juice of 1 lime and a handful of chopped coriander. Season with a pinch of dried chilli flakes and black pepper to taste. Perfect as a dip for vegetables, with salads or with steamed white fish. 4 servings

Fish
and shellfish

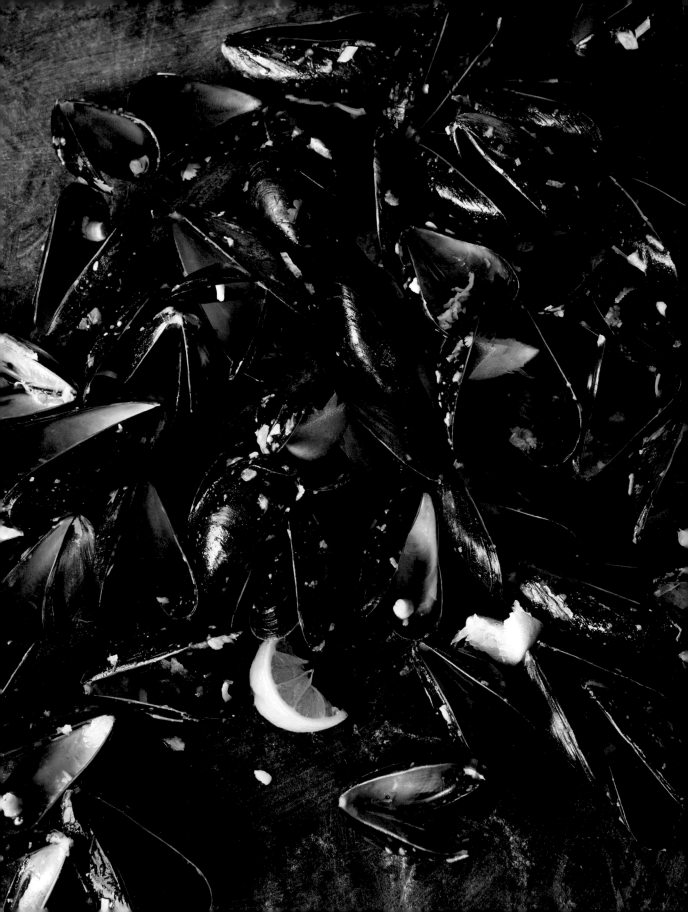

Mussels in a lime, lemongrass and coconut broth

Serves 4

2kg fresh mussels in shells

2 limes

2 lemongrass stalks

1 tsp sunflower oil

2 shallots, peeled and halved

2 garlic cloves, peeled

½ tsp ground turmeric

400ml can light coconut milk

2 tsp maple syrup

2 tsp fish sauce

300g tenderstem broccoli, trimmed

A handful each of coriander and basil leaves, finely chopped, to finish

This deliciously fragrant and light meal will be ready in minutes. Tenderstem broccoli spears are served on the side to dip into the tasty broth.

Scrub the mussels thoroughly under cold running water and remove the hairy beard from the side of the shell. Discard those with broken shells and any that are open and do not close when sharply tapped.

Cut 1 lime into wedges and reserve for serving. Finely zest the other lime and squeeze the juice. Bruise the lemongrass stalks with the back of a knife, remove the coarse outer layers and finely slice the tender inner part.

Put the oil, shallots, garlic, lemongrass slices and turmeric into a small food processor bowl or blender and blitz to a rough paste.

Heat a large pot over a medium-low heat and add the aromatic paste. Cook, stirring, for 2 minutes, until fragrant. Pour in the coconut milk, maple syrup and the lime zest and juice and bring to the boil. Lower the heat and simmer gently for 5 minutes, until slightly reduced. Stir through the fish sauce.

Steam the broccoli for 2–3 minutes, until just tender; keep warm.

Add the mussels to the broth and cover with a tight-fitting lid. Allow the mussels to steam for 4 minutes or until they have opened up; discard any that are still closed.

Using a slotted spoon, divide the mussels between 4 large bowls and pour over the broth. Scatter over the chopped herbs and serve with lime wedges, with the broccoli spears alongside to dip into the broth.

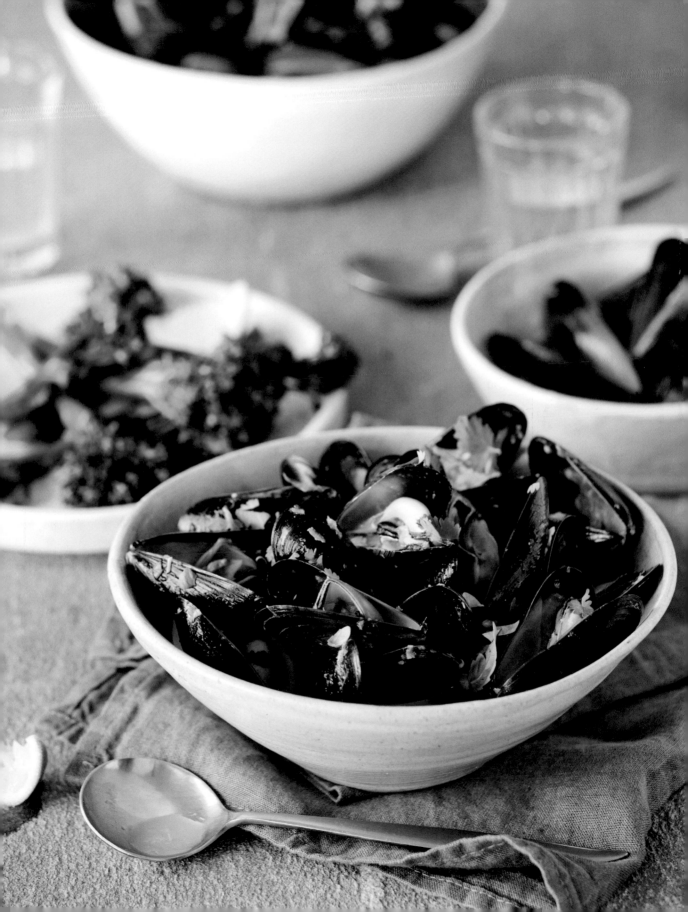

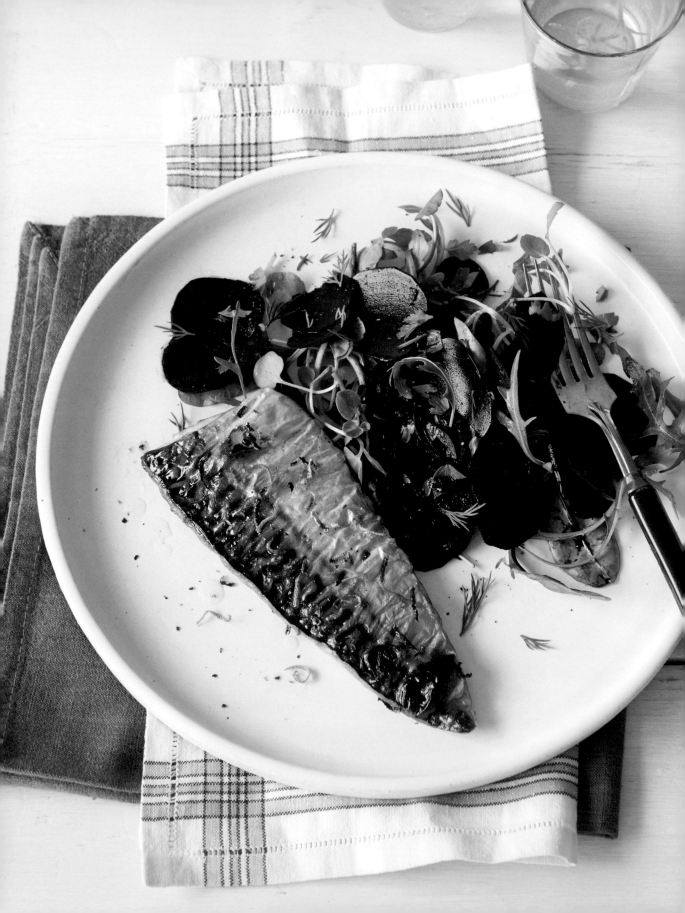

Grilled mackerel with soused beetroot salad

Serves 4

½ red onion, peeled and finely sliced

2 tbsp cider vinegar

Finely grated zest and juice of 2 limes

4 medium raw beetroot

1 tsp maple syrup

A pinch of dried chilli flakes

1 tsp grated horseradish

8 small mackerel fillets

2 tsp light olive oil

A handful of parsley leaves, chopped

2 tbsp dill leaves, chopped

A handful of mixed salad leaves, such as rocket and watercress

Freshly ground black pepper

Mackerel needs to be paired with something that will cut through its oiliness and this briefly soused beetroot salad works perfectly. It doesn't take long for the acidity to permeate the beetroot slices but you can pickle the beetroot up to 2 days ahead for a more pronounced flavour, adding the herbs and leaves just before serving.

Combine the onion, cider vinegar and juice of 1 lime in a bowl and set aside to macerate while you prepare the beetroot.

Peel and slice the beetroot very finely, ideally using a mandoline. Add the beetroot slices, maple syrup, chilli flakes and horseradish to the onion mix and stir to combine. Set aside to pickle slightly.

Preheat the grill to high. Line a grill pan or baking tray with foil and place the mackerel fillets, skin side up, on top. Brush the skin with the olive oil and sprinkle with the zest of 1 lime. Grill for 5 minutes, until the flesh on the underside is opaque and flakes when pressed lightly; the skin should be blistered and charred. Squeeze over the juice and sprinkle with the zest of the remaining lime.

To finish the salad, stir through the parsley, dill and salad leaves and season with black pepper. Serve 2 mackerel fillets per person with a portion of the soused beetroot salad.

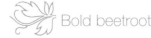 Bold beetroot

This colourful vegetable is delicious eaten raw, finely sliced or shredded. Its vivid purple colour is attributable to betacyanin, a compound shown in research studies to have anti-carcinogenic properties. Beetroot leaves are usually discarded but they can be used like spinach to gain the benefits of their iron and calcium, as well as vitamins A, C and E.

Grilled sardines with salsa verde and quinoa salad

Serves 4

12 sardines, gutted and cleaned

200g quinoa

500ml low-salt vegetable stock

8 sun-dried tomatoes (not in oil)

2 spring onions, finely sliced

2 red chicory bulbs, finely sliced

80g rocket leaves

1 tsp olive oil

Freshly ground black pepper

For the salsa verde

½ garlic clove, peeled

1 tbsp capers, drained

2 tsp Dijon mustard

Juice of 1 lemon

A small handful each of parsley, mint and basil leaves

2 tsp olive oil

3 tbsp water

Sardines are often overlooked but these small oily fish yield so much flavour. A lively salsa verde and a salad alongside turn them into a delicious meal.

Rinse the sardines inside and out and pat dry; set aside.

Put the quinoa in a saucepan, add the stock and bring to a simmer over a medium heat. Simmer for 15 minutes, until the grains are tender and the stock is absorbed, adding a little water if necessary.

Meanwhile put the sun-dried tomatoes into a small bowl and pour on hot water from the kettle to just cover. Leave to rehydrate for 10 minutes, then drain and finely chop the tomatoes.

Transfer the quinoa to a salad bowl and stir through the spring onions, chopped sun-dried tomatoes, chicory and rocket. Drizzle with the olive oil and season with black pepper.

To make the salsa verde, put the garlic, capers, mustard, lemon juice, herbs, olive oil and water in a food processor and blitz until fairly smooth but still retaining a slight texture. The sauce should have the consistency of a pesto; if it is a bit thick, let it down with a little extra water. Set aside whilst you prepare the sardines.

Preheat the grill to high. Lay the sardines on the rack in the grill pan and grill for 2–3 minutes each side, until blistered and tinged with brown; the flesh should come away easily from the bone.

Serve the sardines with the salad and a good dollop of salsa verde.

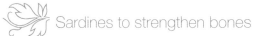 Sardines to strengthen bones

A naturally rich source of dietary vitamin D, sardines provide an excellent and sustainable source of omega-3 rich oily fish in our diets. Their vitamin D content can also promote the growth of healthy bones – a key goal following chemotherapy for all cancer patients.

Grilled tuna with cannellini mash and tomato salsa

Serves 4

4 tuna steaks (about 120g each)

Juice of 1 lemon

1 small red onion, peeled and finely chopped

200g cherry tomatoes, quartered

A handful of basil, roughly chopped

3 tsp olive oil

4 spring onions, sliced

2 garlic cloves, peeled and crushed

2 x 400g cans cannellini beans

120ml low-salt vegetable stock

A small handful of parsley leaves, roughly chopped

Freshly ground black pepper

A couple of cans of cannellini beans are a great standby to have in your storecupboard. They mash beautifully to a creamy textured mash that pairs really well with robust tuna steaks. A quick, zesty salsa brings freshness to this light and satisfying dish.

Have the tuna steaks ready to cook, at room temperature.

To make the salsa, pour half of the lemon juice into a bowl and stir in the red onion. Add the cherry tomatoes and basil and season with black pepper to taste. Set aside whilst you prepare the mash and tuna.

For the mash, heat 2 tsp of the olive oil in a large saucepan over a medium-low heat. When hot, add the spring onions and garlic and fry gently for 2–3 minutes, until softened and golden.

Drain the cannellini beans and add them to the pan. Take off the heat and mash until the beans have broken down to a chunky texture. Pour in the stock and return to the heat for a minute or so to warm through – the mash should be thick and creamy. Add the chopped parsley and the remaining lemon juice and season with pepper to taste. Keep warm.

Heat a non-stick frying pan over a high heat and add the remaining 1 tsp olive oil. When the oil is hot, add the tuna steaks and fry for 2 minutes each side, depending on thickness, turning them once only. The tuna should be pink in the middle.

Remove the tuna steaks from the pan to a warm plate and set aside to rest for a few minutes before serving, with the mash and tomato salsa.

Asian sea bass en papillotte with stir-fried greens

Serves 4

4 sea bass fillets (about 110g each)

3 spring onions, finely sliced

2cm piece of fresh ginger, peeled, finely sliced and cut into fine strips

3 garlic cloves, peeled and finely sliced

1 red chilli, finely sliced, with seeds (optional)

5 tsp low-salt light soy sauce

1 tsp toasted sesame oil

1½ tsp sunflower oil

300g tenderstem broccoli, trimmed

4 tbsp water

1 head of spring greens, roughly sliced

2 tbsp coriander leaves, roughly torn

This dish couldn't be simpler to prepare. Sea bass fillets and aromatics are steamed in little parchment (or foil) tents to condense their delicate flavours and then served with crunchy stir-fried greens.

Preheat the oven to 200°C/Gas 6.

Lay 4 pieces of baking parchment (or foil), each large enough to loosely encase a sea bass fillet, on a work surface. Place a sea bass fillet in the centre of each and sprinkle the spring onions, ginger, one of the sliced garlic cloves, the chilli, 2 tsp of the soy sauce and the sesame oil evenly over the fish.

Bring the edges of the parchment (or foil) up over the fish and fold the edges together well to seal. Transfer to a large baking sheet. Bake for 10–12 minutes until the fish is opaque and flakes easily.

Meanwhile, heat the sunflower oil in a frying pan over a low heat. When it just starts to warm up, add the remaining garlic slices and fry very gently until golden and crisp. Remove the garlic from the pan with a slotted spoon and drain on kitchen paper; set aside.

Place the pan with the garlicky oil back on the hob, over a medium heat. Add the broccoli and water and steam-fry for 4 minutes, until beginning soften. Add the greens and continue to stir-fry for 2–3 minutes until bright green and tender. Stir through the remaining soy sauce.

To serve, carefully unwrap the parcels, retaining all the juices, and sprinkle the torn coriander over the fish. Scatter the fried garlic over the greens and serve with the fish.

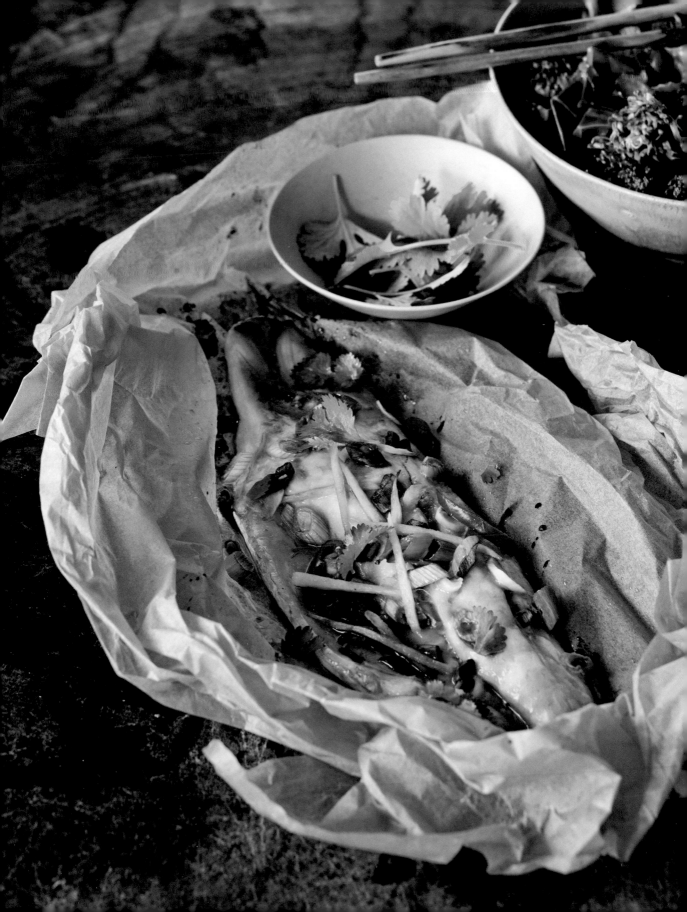

Lemon and almond trout with new potatoes and samphire

Serves 4

4 rainbow trout (about 400g each), gutted and cleaned

400g baby new potatoes, larger ones halved

4 garlic cloves (unpeeled), bashed

3 tsp olive oil

1 lemon, cut into 8 slices

2 tbsp parsley leaves, chopped

1 tbsp tarragon leaves, chopped

2 tbsp flaked almonds

150g samphire, well rinsed

Freshly ground black pepper

This lovely, delicate dish is easy enough to prepare as a midweek dinner yet special enough to serve if you are entertaining.

Preheat the oven to 200°C/Gas 6. Rinse the trout inside and out and pat dry; set aside.

To prepare the potatoes, place them in a large bowl with the garlic, pour over 2 tsp of the olive oil and season with black pepper. Toss to mix, then transfer to a non-stick baking tray. Set aside whilst you prepare the fish.

Lay the trout on a foil-lined baking tray and place 2 slices of lemon in the belly of each. Sprinkle 1 tbsp each of chopped parsley and tarragon evenly over the lemon slices. Brush each trout with a little of the remaining oil and scatter over the almonds.

Bake both the potatoes and trout in the oven for 20–25 minutes, turning the potatoes halfway through cooking, until the trout flesh flakes easily under your fingers when gently pressed and the potatoes are crisp and tender within.

When the trout and potatoes are almost ready, bring a pan of water to the boil. Add the samphire and cook for 1 minute, until just tender, then drain.

Scatter the remaining parsley and tarragon over the trout and serve with the garlicky potatoes and samphire.

Cod with courgettes, peppers and saffron new potatoes

Serves 4

4 cod fillets (about 125g each)

2 tsp olive oil (preferably garlic-flavoured)

2 red peppers, cored, deseeded and roughly sliced

2 medium courgettes, cut into 1cm thick rounds

A pinch of saffron strands

400g new potatoes, larger ones cut in half

2 tsp balsamic vinegar

2 tsp tender rosemary leaves, finely chopped

Freshly ground black pepper

Salad leaves, to serve

It doesn't take many ingredients to make a great meal out of cod – simply roasting chunky fillets with rosemary and vegetables and serving with saffron-infused potatoes makes for a tempting midweek supper.

Have the cod fillets ready to cook, at room temperature. Preheat the oven to 200°C/Gas 6.

Trickle the olive oil into a roasting tin and add the peppers and courgettes. Toss the vegetables so that they are coated in a thin film of oil, season with black pepper and roast in the oven for 12 minutes, until starting to brown at the edges.

Bring a pan of water to the boil, then crumble in the saffron and add the potatoes. Boil for 12–15 minutes, until tender.

Remove the roasting tin from the oven and nestle the cod fillets in amongst the vegetables, skin side down. Drizzle with the balsamic vinegar and brush the fish with the pan juices. Sprinkle with the rosemary and return to the oven for 10–12 minutes, until the cod is opaque and flakes when pressed gently.

Drain the potatoes once they are cooked and keep warm.

Divide the roasted vegetables between warm serving plates and add a cod fillet and a portion of potatoes to each plate. Serve with a scattering of salad leaves.

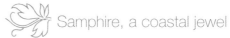 Samphire, a coastal jewel

This succulent seashore plant is rich in a variety of minerals and vitamins A, B and C. With a taste that is naturally salty, it is increasingly favoured as a means of seasoning food negating the need for added salt.

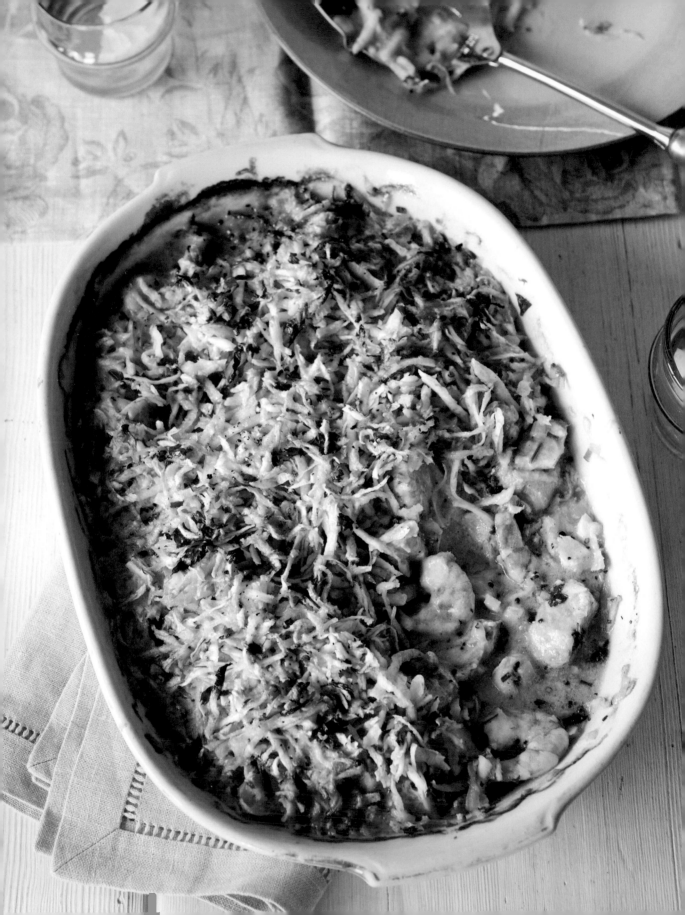

Fish pie
with a celeriac rosti topping

Serves 4

1 tsp sunflower oil

1 small onion, peeled and finely chopped

1 large leek, trimmed, well washed and finely sliced

1 tsp thyme or lemon thyme leaves, roughly chopped

200ml low-salt fish stock

100g low-fat cream cheese

2 tbsp cornflour, mixed with 2 tbsp water

2 tsp wholegrain mustard

250g salmon fillet, skinned and cut into 2cm pieces

150g smoked haddock fillet, skinned and cut into 2cm pieces

200g baby leaf spinach

180g raw king prawns, deveined if necessary

1 tbsp finely chopped chives

2 tbsp chopped parsley leaves

200g peeled celeriac

15g butter, melted

Freshly ground black pepper

A lighter version of the traditional mash-topped family favourite, this recipe is a breeze to prepare and doesn't compromise on flavour. Serve it with seasonal leafy greens or a crisp green salad.

Preheat the oven to 200°C/Gas 6.

Heat the oil in a large, non-stick sauté pan over a medium-low heat. When hot, add the onion, leek and thyme and fry for about 5 minutes, until softened, adding a little water during cooking if the mixture seems dry.

Add the stock, cream cheese and cornflour mixture to the pan and heat, stirring, until thickened, then stir through the mustard. Now add the salmon and haddock pieces and heat very gently for 2 minutes, stirring occasionally and very carefully – so as not to break the pieces up.

Steam the spinach, or cook in a pan with just the water clinging to the leaves after washing, for 1–2 minutes to wilt and then transfer to a sturdy sieve. Press the spinach repeatedly against the sieve to drain off as much water as possible.

When the spinach is fairly dry, pat dry with kitchen paper and lay evenly over the base of a 1.5 litre baking dish.

Carefully stir the prawns, chives and half of the parsley through the fish and spoon on top of the spinach. The sauce will be very thick at this stage but will loosen up as the fish cooks.

Coarsely grate the celeriac and squeeze in your hands to remove as much water as possible. Pat dry with kitchen paper and stir through the melted butter and remaining parsley. Season with black pepper and spoon evenly over the fish.

Bake for 20 minutes, until bubbling around the edges and the topping is crisp and golden. If the top appears to be colouring too quickly in the oven, cover loosely with foil.

Almond-crusted cod with tomato beans

Serves 4

50g raw almonds

2 tsp wholegrain mustard

1 tbsp parsley leaves

1 tbsp basil leaves

Finely grated zest of 1 lemon

4 cod fillets (about 125g each)

1 egg white, lightly beaten

2 tsp olive oil

300g fine green beans, trimmed

1 garlic clove, peeled and crushed

½ tsp paprika

200g cherry tomatoes, halved

2 tsp tomato purée

4 tbsp water

Freshly ground black pepper

Lemon wedges, to serve

Sweet almonds and vibrant herbs are blitzed together to make a tasty, crunchy topping for mild, chunky cod fillets. Tender green beans in a rich tomato sauce are the perfect complement for this easy-to-prepare supper.

Preheat the oven to 200°C/Gas 6.

Put the almonds, mustard, parsley, basil and lemon zest in a small food processor bowl and season with black pepper. Pulse until the almonds have broken down to resemble coarse breadcrumbs.

Brush each of the cod fillets with a little egg white and sprinkle the almond mixture on top of them, pressing it down to adhere. Place the cod fillets on a non-stick baking tray and bake for 10–12 minutes, until the topping is crisp and golden and the fish flakes when lightly pressed.

Meanwhile, heat the olive oil in a large sauté pan over a medium heat. When hot, add the beans and fry for 2 minutes, then add the garlic, paprika, cherry tomatoes and tomato purée. Fry, stirring for a minute, until fragrant. Add the water and continue to cook for a further 1–2 minutes, until the beans are tender but still vibrant green and the tomatoes have broken down.

Serve the baked cod with the tomato beans and lemon wedges for squeezing.

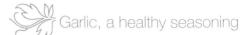 Garlic, a healthy seasoning

Treatments for cancer have a profound effect on our natural immunity. Recent studies suggest that including garlic in our diets may provide a means of redressing this naturally. Further research is needed to verify this, but garlic is known to possess many other health benefits, including vitamins C and B6, selenium and other antioxidants, including allicin. In a healthy diet, it is particularly valuable as a flavouring alternative to salt.

Roasted spiced monkfish
with tomatoes and chicory

Serves 4

500g monkfish tail fillet

2 tsp ground cumin

1 tsp ground coriander

1 tsp ground turmeric

1 tsp garam masala

2 tsp vegetable oil

2 chicory bulbs, quartered
lengthways

200g cherry tomatoes

1 garlic clove, peeled and
crushed

2cm piece of fresh ginger, peeled
and finely grated

300g asparagus spears

2 tsp tamarind paste

Juice of ½ pink grapefruit

1 tbsp coriander leaves

The meaty robustness of monkfish ensures it holds its own when teamed with intense flavours. The sweetness of the fish works brilliantly here with aromatic spices and a rich, tangy dressing.

Preheat the oven to 200°C/Gas 6. Remove any grey sinew still attached to the monkfish, using a small knife.

In a small bowl, mix together the ground spices. Spoon half of this mixture into a large bowl and stir in the oil. Add the chicory and tomatoes to the bowl and toss to coat them in the oily spices, then transfer to a non-stick roasting tray; save the spicy oil remaining in the bowl. Roast in the oven for 8 minutes.

Meanwhile, add the garlic, ginger and remaining ground spices to the bowl (used to toss the chicory and tomatoes). Now add the monkfish and rub the spices and aromatics all over the flesh.

Snap off the woody ends of the asparagus spears.

After the 8 minutes' roasting, take the roasting tray from the oven and tuck the monkfish in amongst the vegetables. Quickly toss the asparagus in any remaining spices and oil in the bowl, add to the tray and return to the oven.

Roast for 10 minutes, or until the monkfish is cooked through and tender in the centre; do not overcook, or the flesh will toughen. Remove from the oven and set aside to rest for a few minutes.

Meanwhile, for the dressing, mix together the tamarind paste, grapefruit juice and coriander.

To serve, cut the monkfish into slices and serve on a bed of the vegetables, with the dressing trickled on top.

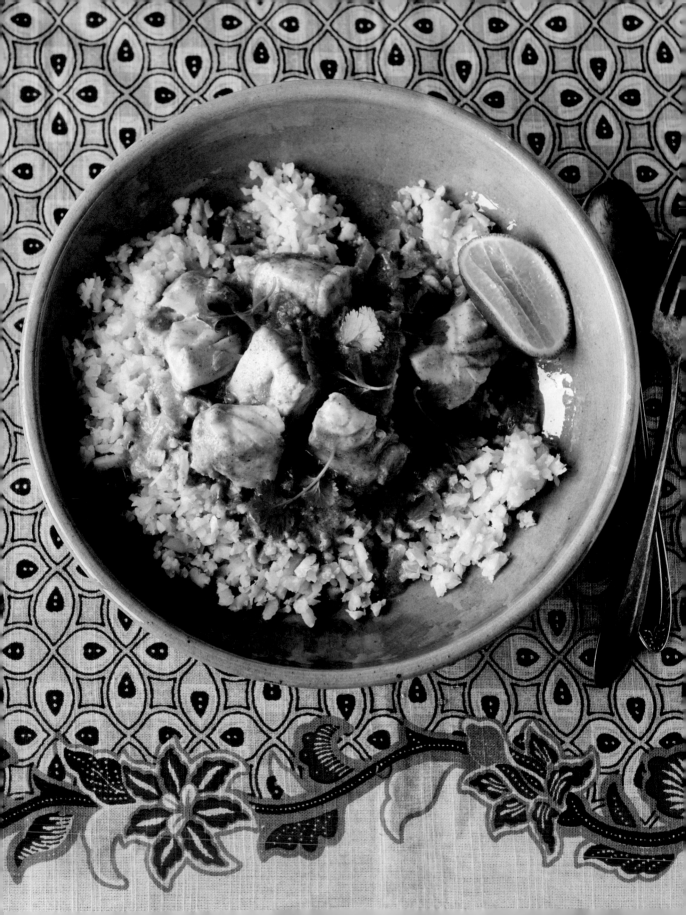

Coconut fish curry with cauliflower 'rice'

Serves 4

500g cod fillet

2 tsp sunflower oil

1 onion, peeled and finely chopped

2cm piece of fresh ginger, peeled and finely grated

1 tsp each of ground coriander, cumin and turmeric

2 tsp tamarind paste

400ml can coconut milk

1 low-salt fish stock cube

A pinch of dried chilli flakes (optional)

1 medium cauliflower

A handful of coriander leaves

Lime wedges, to serve

This gently spiced curry, served with steamed cauliflower blitzed to resemble fluffy rice grains, makes for a lovely, comforting supper.

Cut the cod into 4cm chunks and set aside.

Heat the oil in a large, deep frying pan or sauté pan over a medium-low heat. When hot, add the onion and fry gently for 5 minutes or until softened, adding a little water if it seems dry. Stir through the ginger and ground spices and fry for 2 minutes, until fragrant.

Stir in the tamarind paste and coconut milk, then crumble in the stock cube and add the chilli flakes, if using. Simmer for 5 minutes to reduce slightly.

To make the cauliflower 'rice', cut the cauliflower into florets and steam for 2–3 minutes, until just tender. Allow to steam-dry off the heat, then tip into a food processor and pulse to break up into rice-like 'grains' (alternatively you can coarsely grate the cauliflower). Keep warm.

Add the pieces of cod to the curry sauce and simmer gently for 2 minutes, being careful not to break the fish up. The fish is ready when it is opaque and flakes when pressed gently.

Serve the curry and cauliflower 'rice' scattered with coriander, with a wedge of lime for squeezing.

Fish tagine with herbed bulgar wheat

Serves 4

500g firm white fish fillet, such as haddock, pollack or cod

2 tsp olive oil

1 onion, peeled and finely chopped

2 garlic cloves, peeled and crushed

2cm piece of fresh ginger, peeled and finely grated

2 tsp ground cumin

1 tsp ground coriander

1 tsp ground turmeric

A pinch of dried chilli flakes (optional)

2 tsp tomato purée

A pinch of saffron strands

500ml low-salt fish stock

400g tomatoes, roughly chopped

Finely grated zest and juice of 2 clementines

200g bulgar wheat, well rinsed

600ml water

A small handful each of mint, parsley and coriander leaves, roughly chopped

This gently spiced dish is so easy and quick to prepare. To make it even faster to serve up, you can make the sauce the day before, or well in advance and freeze it; simply defrost, bring up to heat and add the fish at the last minute.

Cut the white fish into 4cm pieces and set aside.

Heat the olive oil in a large sauté pan or flameproof casserole over a medium-low heat. When hot, add the onion and fry gently for about 5 minutes until softened, adding a little water if it seems a bit dry. Add the garlic, ginger, cumin, coriander, turmeric, chilli flakes if using, and the tomato purée. Cook for 2 minutes, stirring frequently, until fragrant.

Crumble the saffron strands into the stock and add to the pan, along with the chopped tomatoes and the clementine zest and juice. Simmer for 10 minutes, until slightly reduced.

Meanwhile, tip the bulgar wheat into a separate pan, pour on the water and bring to a simmer. Lower the heat and simmer for 12–15 minutes or until the water has been absorbed and the grains are tender, adding a little more water if necessary during cooking.

Add the chunks of fish to the tagine and simmer very gently for 2 minutes, until opaque and flaking to the touch. Be careful not to break the fish up by stirring.

Toss the chopped herbs through the cooked bulgar wheat and serve with the tagine.

Salmon is a good source of omega-3 fatty acids, which play an important role in health. Thought to reduce inflammation and lower blood pressure, they may also be natural chemo-preventive agents that can inhibit or impede cancer. These recipe ideas will tempt you towards the recommended one or two oily fish portions each week. Each serves 4.

Baked salmon with avocado and radish salad

Brush 4 salmon fillets with 1 tsp olive oil and sprinkle with the grated zest of 1 lime. Bake at 200°C/Gas 6 for 10–12 minutes. Meanwhile, toss 1 sliced avocado with 100g sliced radishes, ½ sliced cucumber and a handful of torn coriander leaves. Dress with 2 tsp low-salt soy sauce mixed with the juice of 1 lime. Serve the salad with the salmon fillets.

Grilled salmon with grilled peaches and ginger

Heat a griddle pan over a high heat. Finely grate a 2cm piece of fresh ginger. Rub 4 salmon fillets and 4 halved peaches with the grated ginger and 2 tsp olive oil. Griddle for 6 minutes until the salmon is just cooked and the peaches are syrupy. Serve with lemon wedges and rocket.

Salmon skewers with a lime and ginger dressing

Cut 4 salmon fillets into chunks and thread onto 8 skewers. Mix 15g melted butter with 2cm finely grated ginger and the juice of 1 lime. Brush the skewers with some of the flavoured butter and grill for 6 minutes. Meanwhile, toss 2 grated carrots, ½ sliced red cabbage and 4 spring onions together with the juice of 1 lime and a handful of torn coriander. Brush the grilled salmon with the remaining butter and serve with the salad.

Poached salmon, pea and broad bean salad

Flake 4 poached salmon fillets and toss with 200g each of blanched peas and broad beans, a handful of rocket, the finely grated zest and juice of 1 lemon, a handful of chopped parsley and 20g crumbled light feta.

Sesame-crusted salmon with pak choi

Mix 2 tbsp sesame seeds with 2 tsp low-salt soy sauce and 1 tsp clear honey. Spread evenly over 4 salmon fillets and bake at 200°C/Gas 6 for 10–12 minutes. Serve the salmon with the pan juices spooned over and steamed pak choi on the side.

Poultry
and meat

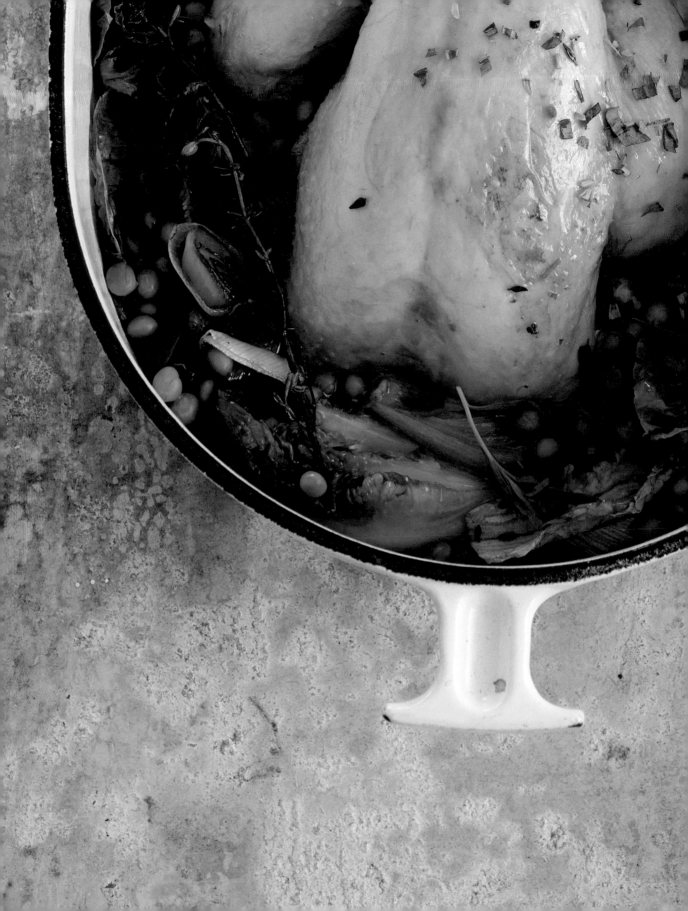

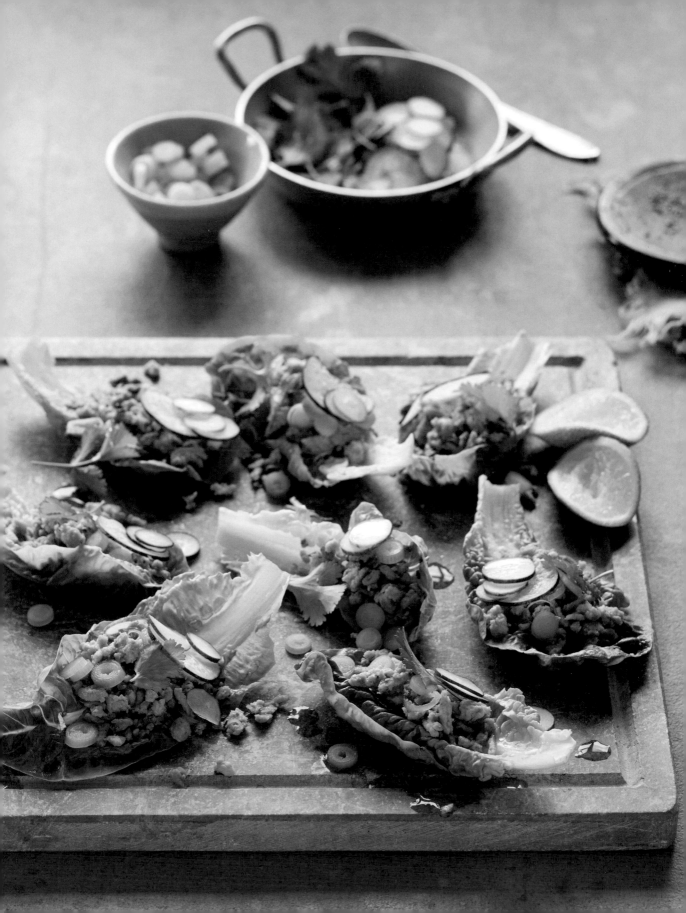

Thai turkey lettuce cups

Serves 4

1 lemongrass stalk

2 tsp sunflower oil

500g lean turkey mince (breast)

Juice of 1 lime

2 tsp fish sauce

3 tsp maple syrup

A pinch of dried chilli flakes (optional)

4 Little Gem lettuces, leaves separated

100g radishes, sliced

4 spring onions, finely sliced

A small handful of coriander leaves, roughly chopped

Full of vibrant Thai flavours, these protein-packed lettuce cups are perfect for a light, fresh-tasting supper, and they can be prepared in minutes.

Bruise the lemongrass stalk with the flat of a knife, remove the tough outer layers and finely slice the tender inner part.

Heat half the oil in a large frying pan over a medium heat. When hot, add half of the turkey mince, along with the sliced lemongrass. Fry for 4–5 minutes until golden brown, breaking up the mince into small pieces with a wooden spoon as you go. Remove from the pan and repeat with the remaining oil and turkey mince.

In a small bowl, stir together the lime juice, fish sauce, maple syrup and chilli flakes, if using.

Return all the cooked mince to the pan, add the lime and fish sauce mixture and stir to combine. Cook over a high heat for 2–3 minutes, until the turkey is completely cooked through and the mixture is golden brown and sticky.

Spoon the hot mince into the lettuce leaves (or onto a platter lined with the lettuce so that everyone can help themselves). Scatter over the radish slices, spring onions and coriander and enjoy.

Warm chicken liver salad

Serves 4

100g asparagus

100g fine green beans, trimmed

2 tsp olive oil

400g chicken livers, trimmed
and patted dry

1 tsp paprika

1 chicory bulb, leaves separated

100g cherry tomatoes, halved

A handful of rocket leaves

Juice of 1 lemon, or to taste

Freshly ground black pepper

Tender and flavoursome, chicken livers offer so much
more than a base for pâtés and terrines. Teaming them
with a little paprika and bittersweet salad ingredients
creates a dish that sings with texture and taste.

Snap off the woody ends of the asparagus and cut the spears into
2–3cm pieces. Cut the green beans in half. Bring a pan of water
to the boil. Add the asparagus and beans, bring back to a simmer
and cook for 2–3 minutes until just tender. Drain and set aside.

Heat the olive oil in a large, non-stick frying pan. Toss the chicken
livers in the paprika and add to the hot pan. Fry for 5–7 minutes,
turning every so often, until golden but still a little pink within.

Toss the warm chicken livers with the asparagus and beans,
chicory, tomatoes and rocket. Add the lemon juice and season
with black pepper to taste. Serve immediately.

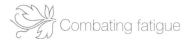 Combating fatigue

Tiredness is a common consequence of cancer
treatments and for anyone with rheumatoid arthritis
the impact can be worsened by iron-deficiency
anaemia, which reduces the amount of oxygen that
can be carried by the blood. Offal, such as liver and
kidneys, are a concentrated source of iron, which can
alleviate such concerns relatively quickly to enable
you to get back on your feet.

Turkey and pearl barley risotto with tarragon

Serves 4

2 tsp olive oil

1 small onion, peeled and finely diced

1 leek, trimmed, well washed and finely sliced

2 garlic cloves, peeled and crushed

250g lean turkey mince

200g pearl barley

About 1.2 litres hot low-salt chicken stock

2 thyme sprigs

150g frozen peas

Finely grated zest of ½ lemon

1–2 tbsp tarragon leaves, roughly chopped

20g Parmesan, finely grated (optional)

Freshly ground black pepper

Pearl barley offers a wholesome alternative to risotto rice in this soothing, one-pan supper. Tarragon lends a distinctive flavour but you could use thyme or parsley if you prefer.

Heat the olive oil in a large, non-stick sauté pan over a medium-low heat. When it is hot, add the onion and leek to the pan and fry gently for about 5 minutes until softened and golden, adding a little splash of water if it seems a bit dry. Add the garlic and fry for a further minute.

Now add the turkey mince, turning up the heat slightly. Fry the mince, breaking it up with a wooden spoon, for 2–3 minutes until nicely golden. Tip in the pearl barley and fry for another minute.

Pour over 800ml of the stock, add the thyme and bring to the boil. Lower the heat and simmer gently for 35–40 minutes until the barley is tender, topping up with more stock during cooking if the mixture is looking a little dry, and adding the peas for the last minute of cooking.

Remove the pan from the heat and add the grated lemon zest, chopped tarragon and Parmesan, if using. Season with black pepper and serve.

Pot-roast chicken
with braised lettuce and peas

Serves 4–6

2 tsp olive oil

200g shallots, peeled and halved if large

2 leeks, trimmed, well washed and roughly sliced

4 garlic cloves, peeled and crushed

2 generous thyme sprigs

2 bay leaves

1 oven-ready free-range chicken (about 1.5kg)

400ml low-salt chicken stock

4 Little Gem lettuces, halved lengthways

350g frozen petits pois

2 tsp chopped tarragon or chervil

A squeeze of lemon juice

Freshly ground black pepper

It takes very few ingredients to turn a good quality, whole chicken into a tempting meal. This slow-cooked one-pot chicken is simplicity itself – perfect for an effortless light Sunday lunch.

Preheat the oven to 140°C/Gas 1.

Heat the olive oil a large flameproof casserole (big enough to comfortably hold the whole chicken) over a medium heat. When the oil is hot, add the shallots and leeks and fry gently, turning occasionally, for 5 minutes or until lightly coloured and softened. Add the garlic, thyme and bay leaves and fry for a further minute, until fragrant.

Add the whole chicken to the dish and nestle it in amongst the vegetables, then pour over the stock. Bring to simmering point, then cover the dish tightly with a lid or foil and transfer to the oven. Cook for 1½ hours, basting the chicken with the pan juices occasionally.

Now turn the oven setting up to 190°C/Gas 5 and uncover the dish. Roast, uncovered, for a further 15 minutes, adding the lettuce and petits pois 5 minutes before the end of cooking. By now the chicken should be tender and cooked through with golden skin. The vegetables should be just tender.

Stir in the tarragon or chervil and finish with a squeeze of lemon juice and a sprinkling of black pepper.

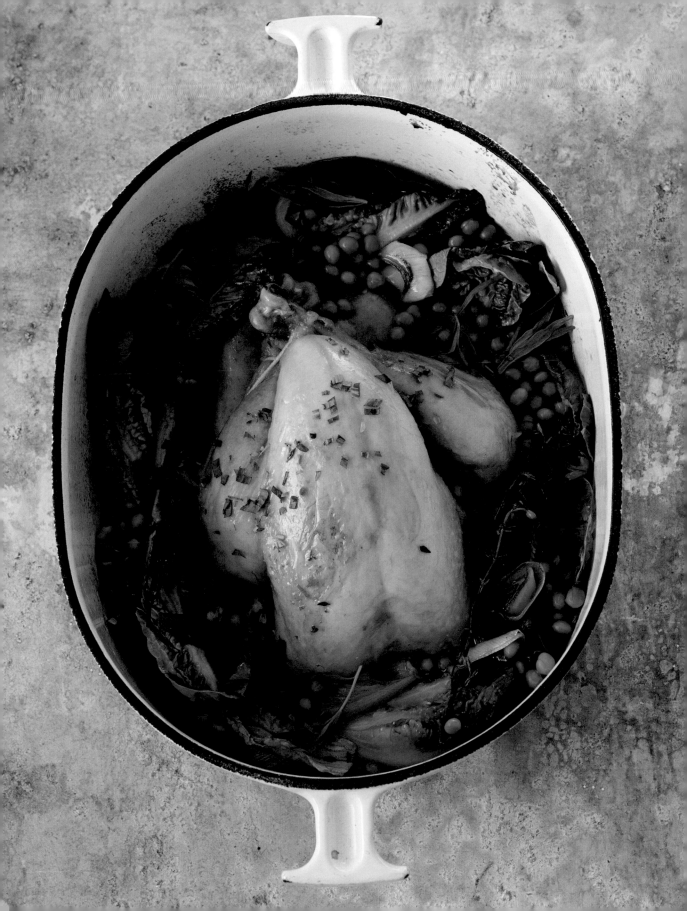

Paprika-roast chicken with sweet potatoes and red cabbage slaw

Serves 4

1 oven-ready free-range chicken (about 1.5kg)

1 lemon

2 tsp smoked paprika

2 tsp olive oil

1 tsp clear honey

2 garlic cloves, peeled and bashed

A few thyme sprigs

1 onion, peeled and cut into thick slices

800g sweet potatoes, scrubbed and cut into wedges

For the red cabbage slaw

½ red cabbage, shredded

4 spring onions, sliced

2 carrots, peeled and coarsely grated

4 radishes, finely sliced

2 tbsp chives, roughly chopped

2 tbsp low-fat natural yogurt

Juice of 1 lime

For Sunday lunch with a difference, try this tasty roast chicken with its sweet and smoky flavours. Teamed with roasted sweet potato wedges and red cabbage slaw it's a mouth-watering assembly.

Preheat the oven to 200°C/Gas 6.

Place the chicken on a board. Squeeze the juice from the lemon and mix with the paprika, olive oil and honey. Spread half of this mixture over the chicken. Put the lemon shells, garlic cloves and thyme sprigs into the cavity.

Lay the onion slices over the base of a non-stick roasting tin and place the chicken on top. Roast for 20 minutes, then turn the heat down to 180°C/Gas 4 and roast for a further 15 minutes.

Now toss the sweet potato wedges in the remaining paprika mix and place them around the chicken. (If you are short on space, put the potato wedges in a separate roasting tin.) Roast for a further 30–45 minutes, basting occasionally and turning the sweet potatoes, until the chicken is cooked through and tender.

Meanwhile, to make the slaw, simply toss together the cabbage, spring onions, carrots, radishes and chives together in a bowl. Mix the yogurt with the lime juice and use to dress the slaw.

Remove the chicken from the oven and leave to rest in a warm place for about 10 minutes before carving; keep the sweet potatoes warm.

Carve the chicken and serve with the sweet potato wedges and red cabbage slaw.

Sesame beef skewers with stir-fried rainbow vegetables

Serves 4

560g lean rump or other steak

2 tsp toasted sesame oil

2.5cm piece of fresh ginger, peeled and finely grated

3 garlic cloves, peeled and crushed

2 tsp maple syrup

4 tsp low-salt soy sauce

1 tsp sesame seeds

2 carrots

1 red pepper, cored, deseeded and sliced

200g broccoli, cut into bite-sized florets

4 spring onions, finely sliced

150g sugar snap peas

Lime wedges, to serve

Bright, colourful and full of aromatic flavours, this combination will liven up the dullest of days.

Cut the steak into 24 cubes and place in a non-metallic bowl. Spoon over half the sesame oil, 2 crushed garlic cloves, the ginger, maple syrup, soy sauce and sesame seeds. Stir to combine and set aside for at least 10 minutes, or up to overnight in the fridge.

Using a vegetable peeler, cut the carrots lengthways into long ribbons and place in a bowl.

Heat the grill to high. Thread 3 cubes of meat onto each of 8 metal skewers and lay on a grill tray. Reserve the marinade. Grill for 3–4 minutes, turning once, until browned but still pink in the middle.

Meanwhile, heat a wok or non-stick frying pan over a medium heat. Add the remaining sesame oil. When hot, add the red pepper and broccoli and stir-fry for 2 minutes. Add the remaining garlic and the spring onions and cook for a further minute.

Pour in the remaining marinade and toss in the carrot ribbons and sugar snaps. Stir-fry for another minute or two until the vegetables are tender but still crisp. Serve 2 skewers per person with the stir-fried veg and a wedge of lime.

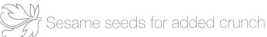 Sesame seeds for added crunch

These nutrient-packed seeds are used extensively in Middle Eastern and Asian cookery, either plain or toasted, and as sesame oil and tahini paste. An excellent source of minerals, they are also among the most abundant dietary source of plant lignans, which are known to hinder the production and spread of certain tumour cells. Toasted sesame seeds are an effective seasoning and textural contrast for salads and other dishes.

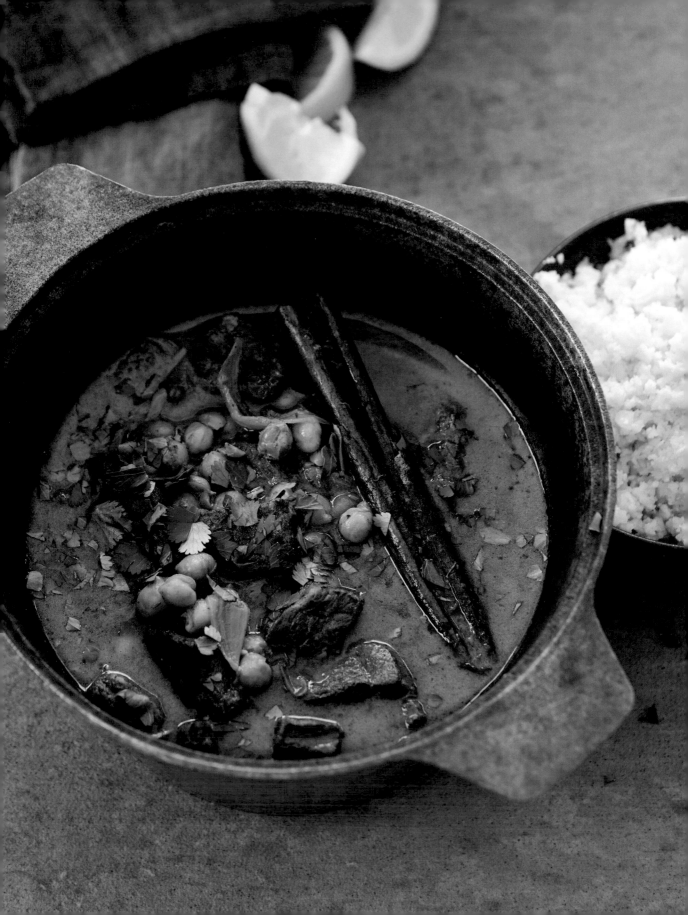

Fragrant braised beef with dates and chickpeas

Serves 4

2 tsp olive oil

560g lean beef stewing steak, cut into 2.5cm cubes

6 tbsp water

1 large onion, peeled and roughly sliced

4 garlic cloves, peeled and crushed

2.5cm piece of fresh ginger, peeled and grated

1 cinnamon stick

2 tsp ground cumin

A pinch of saffron strands

650ml hot low-salt beef stock

75g Medjool dates, pitted and sliced in half

400g can chickpeas, drained

1 medium cauliflower

A small handful each of coriander and parsley leaves, roughly chopped

Lemon wedges, to serve

A lighter take on a traditional Moroccan tagine, this mildly spiced braise is warming, aromatic and deeply comforting. Served with cauliflower 'rice', it's perfect for supper on a chilly winter's evening.

Preheat the oven to 140°C/Gas 1.

Heat 1 tsp of the olive oil in a large, non-stick frying pan over a medium-high heat. When hot, brown the cubes of meat, turning occasionally, for 3–4 minutes until well coloured all over; you may need to do this in two batches to avoid overcrowding the pan.

Transfer the beef to a casserole dish (or tagine). Add 3 tbsp of the water to the frying pan and swirl it around, scraping up any meaty residue. Pour this deglazing liquor into the casserole.

Heat the remaining oil in the frying pan. Once hot, fry the onion slices for 2–3 minutes, turning every so often, until golden. Add the garlic, ginger, cinnamon, cumin and saffron to the pan and fry for a further minute or so, until fragrant. Scrape the onion and spice mixture into the casserole, then deglaze the pan again with the remaining 3 tbsp water.

Pour over the stock, ensuring the meat is just covered, adding a little more if necessary. Stir in the dates, then cover the casserole with a lid and transfer to the oven. Braise for 1 hour, then take out the casserole and stir in the chickpeas. Return to the oven for a further 1½ hours or until the meat is tender.

To make the cauliflower 'rice', cut the cauliflower into florets and steam for 2–3 minutes, until just tender. Allow to steam-dry off the heat, then tip into a food processor and pulse to break up into rice-like 'grains' (alternatively you can coarsely grate the cauli).

Serve the beef with the cauliflower 'rice', topped with a scattering of coriander and with lemon wedges on the side.

Harissa lamb with griddled vegetables and a tahini dressing

Serves 4

500g lamb neck fillets, trimmed of any excess fat

1 tbsp good quality harissa paste, such as Belazu

2 garlic cloves, peeled and crushed

Finely grated zest and juice of 1 lemon

2 courgettes

1 fennel bulb

1 medium aubergine

2 red peppers, halved, cored and deseeded

1–2 tsp olive oil

2 tbsp tahini

4 tbsp water

A small handful of flat-leaf parsley leaves

Tender neck of lamb is inexpensive and perfect for quick cooking. This spicy, Middle Eastern inspired dish is a cinch to prepare and impressive enough to serve if you are entertaining.

Preheat the oven to 200°C/Gas 6.

Place the lamb neck fillets in a non-metallic bowl and add the harissa, 1 crushed garlic clove and half of the lemon zest and juice. Toss well to coat the lamb and set aside for 5 minutes – or leave overnight in the fridge if you want to prepare ahead.

Cut the courgettes, fennel and aubergine into 1cm thick slices; cut each of the pepper halves into 4 wedges. Heat a large griddle pan over a high heat. While it is heating, brush the vegetable slices with the olive oil.

Once the griddle is smoking hot, add the lamb and griddle, turning occasionally, for 3–4 minutes to brown. Transfer the browned lamb to a baking sheet and roast in the oven for 15 minutes for medium pinkness, 20 minutes for well done.

While the lamb is in the oven, griddle the vegetables in batches for 1–2 minutes each side, until tender and tinged with brown. Once cooked, lay them out flat on a baking sheet (as piling them up would cause them to steam and overcook).

Whisk together the remaining garlic, lemon zest and juice, the tahini and water to make a dressing.

When the lamb is cooked, set it aside to rest for up to 10 minutes before slicing and tossing with the griddled vegetables. Serve drizzled with the dressing and scattered with chopped parsley.

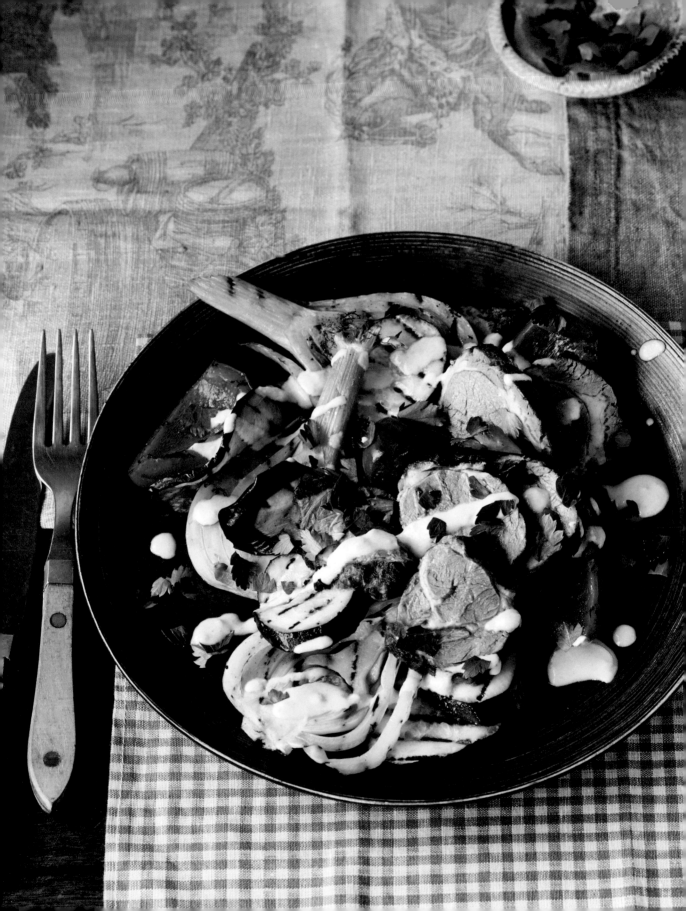

Pistachio-crusted lamb fillets with roasted pepper salad

Serves 4

3 tsp olive oil

500g lamb neck fillets, trimmed of any excess fat

50g shelled, unroasted and unsalted pistachio nuts

3 tbsp flat-leaf parsley leaves

1 tbsp tender rosemary leaves

1 fat garlic clove, peeled

Finely grated zest of ½ lemon

1 red pepper, cored, deseeded and sliced

1 green pepper, cored, deseeded and sliced

1 yellow pepper, cored, deseeded and sliced

½ red onion, peeled and finely sliced

½ tsp caraway seeds

1 tbsp cider vinegar

Sweet and vibrantly green, pistachios complement this delicate cut of lamb perfectly. Easy to prepare and quick to roast, the crusted lamb is served with a lovely, textured roasted pepper salad.

Preheat the oven to 200°C/Gas 6.

Heat 1 tsp of the olive oil in a large, non-stick frying pan. When hot, add the lamb neck fillets and fry for 3–4 minutes, turning occasionally, until golden brown all over. Remove from the pan and set aside on a board to cool slightly.

Meanwhile, tip the pistachios, 1 tbsp of the parsley, the rosemary, garlic and lemon zest into a food processor and pulse until the mixture resembles fine breadcrumbs.

Divide the pistachio crumb mixture between the lamb fillets and, using your fingers, pack a layer on top of each fillet to create a crust. Place the fillets in a roasting tray and roast in the oven for 15 minutes for medium pinkness, 20 minutes for well done.

While the lamb is cooking, toss the peppers in the remaining olive oil with the onion and caraway seeds and roast on a separate baking tray in the oven for 10–15 minutes, until tinged with brown but still with a crunch.

Allow the lamb to rest in a warm place for 10 minutes before serving. Toss the roasted peppers with the cider vinegar and remaining parsley. Cut the lamb into slices and serve with the roasted pepper salad.

Lamb's liver with sage and wild mushrooms

Serves 4

450g lamb's liver, sliced

2 tbsp plain flour

2 tsp sunflower oil

2 shallots, peeled and finely sliced

2 garlic cloves, peeled and finely sliced

250g wild mushrooms, wiped clean

8 sage leaves, roughly chopped

250ml hot low-salt lamb stock

A splash of Worcestershire sauce

100g rocket, spinach and watercress leaves

Freshly ground black pepper

Lemon wedges, to serve

Golden and crisp on the outside and meltingly tender within, fried lamb's liver is very good when it's properly cooked. Here wild mushrooms and sage bring out the savoury earthiness of this often-overlooked cut.

Rinse the lamb's liver in a colander under cold water and pat dry with kitchen paper. Season the flour generously with pepper and dust the liver with the seasoned flour.

Heat half of the oil in a large, non-stick frying pan over a medium heat. When hot, add half of the liver slices to the pan and fry for 3–4 minutes, turning occasionally, until well browned. Set the browned liver aside on a plate and repeat with the remaining liver.

Heat the remaining oil in the frying pan. Add the shallots, garlic, mushrooms and sage leaves and fry for 2–3 minutes until golden. Remove from the pan and set aside on a plate.

Pour the stock into the pan and simmer to reduce slightly. Return the liver to the pan and simmer very gently for a minute or two. Return the mushroom mixture to the pan, add the Worcestershire sauce and toss to combine.

Serve at once, with the salad leaves and lemon wedges.

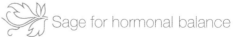 Sage for hormonal balance

Historically, sage has been used medicinally to alleviate a range of ailments, including digestive problems, menopausal symptoms and loss of memory. It was even a component of a medicine used to ward off the plague! Rich in phytochemicals and a good source of vital nutrients, including vitamins A, C and K and several B vitamins, as well as important minerals, it offers health benefits, but a complex interplay of processes is likely to explain such effects.

It is thought that sage's phytochemical content may prevent the formation, block the action and/or suppress the development of cancer from carcinogens.

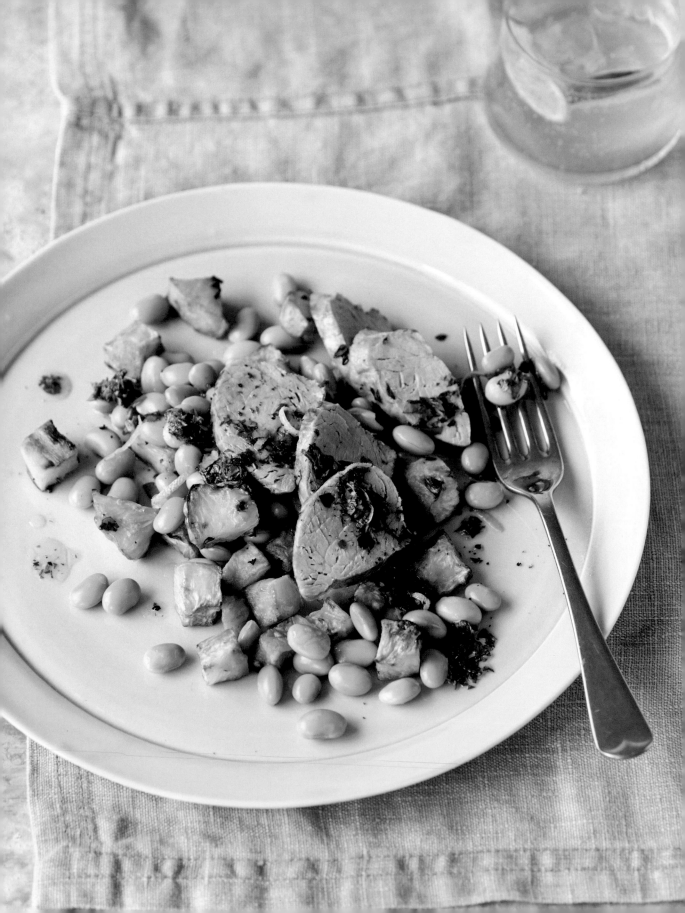

Roasted pork tenderloin with celeriac, edamame beans and gremolata

Serves 4

3 tsp olive oil

1 medium celeriac, peeled and cut into 1.5cm cubes

1 pork tenderloin, trimmed of excess fat and sinew

1 tsp thyme leaves, roughly chopped

Finely grated zest and juice of ½ lemon

1 small garlic clove, peeled and crushed

4 tbsp flat-leaf parsley leaves, finely chopped

A pinch of mineral salt

1–2 tbsp water

200g frozen edamame beans

Edamame – nutritious young green soy beans – and celeriac team nicely with roasted pork tenderloin, and a zesty gremolata marries the flavours together nicely.

Preheat the oven to 200°C/Gas 6.

Spoon 1 tsp of the olive oil into a large bowl and tumble in the celeriac. Stir to give it a fine coating of oil and spread out on a baking tray in a single layer (use two trays if necessary). Roast in the oven for 10 minutes.

Meanwhile, heat a non-stick frying pan over a medium heat and add ½ tsp olive oil. When hot, add the pork tenderloin and fry for 3–4 minutes, turning occasionally, until golden brown all over. Remove the pork from the pan.

Take the baking tray out of the oven and lay the pork tenderloin on top of the celeriac. Sprinkle with the thyme and return to the oven. Roast for a further 25–30 minutes until cooked through.

Whilst the pork is in the oven, prepare the gremolata. Simply stir together the remaining 1½ tsp olive oil, the lemon zest and juice, garlic, parsley and salt and mix in 1–2 tbsp water to loosen the consistency to your liking.

Once the pork is cooked, rest in a warm place for 5 minutes or so. Add the edamame beans to a pan of boiling water and simmer for about 3 minutes until tender but still with a slight bite. Drain well.

Slice the pork and serve with the celeriac, beans and gremolata.

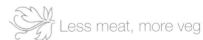 Less meat, more veg

Combining meat with soy-rich edamame beans is a great way to maximise the nutritional value of a meal. Pork is a good source of protein and iron to combat lethargy, while edamame beans are low in fat and high in protein, fibre and a host of other vitamins and minerals – a real nutritional powerhouse.

Venison and chestnut stew with pearl barley

Serves 4–6

2 tsp sunflower or vegetable oil

500g venison shoulder, diced into 2.5cm pieces

About 1 litre low-salt beef stock

1 large onion, peeled and roughly sliced

200g carrots, peeled and roughly chopped

2 garlic cloves, peeled and crushed

100g pearl barley

1 tbsp tomato purée

A few thyme sprigs

2 bay leaves

200g vacuum-packed chestnuts

125g chestnut mushrooms, halved

200g kale, shredded

Juice of ½ lemon

This stew brings together some of the best flavours of the colder months. The rich, gamey flavour of venison is mellowed with winter vegetables and wholesome pearl barley. Bright, lemony kale cuts through the richness.

Preheat the oven to 140°C/Gas 1.

Heat half of the oil in a large non-stick frying pan over a medium heat. When hot, add the pieces of venison and fry until golden brown on all sides; you may need to do this in two batches to avoid overcrowding the pan. Remove the venison from the pan and transfer to a large flameproof casserole.

Pour a little of the stock into the hot pan and swirl around, scraping up any residue. Pour this deglazing liquor into the casserole. Wipe out the frying pan.

Heat a little more oil in the frying pan and fry the onion and carrots until golden. Transfer the veg to the casserole and deglaze the pan as above, adding the liquor to the casserole. Finish by frying the garlic in the last of the oil and adding it to the casserole.

Add the pearl barley to the casserole and pour on enough of the remaining stock to just cover everything. Stir in the tomato purée and add the thyme and bay leaves. Place over a medium heat and bring the stew to a simmer. Lay a damp piece of greaseproof paper directly on the surface, cover with a lid and cook in the oven for 1 hour.

Take the casserole from the oven and stir in the chestnuts and mushrooms. If the stew is looking a little dry at this stage, add up to 250ml more stock (or water). Return the casserole to the oven for another hour.

By this stage, the stew should be rich and unctuous, with a fairly thick sauce – thin it a little with water if you wish. The venison should be meltingly tender – if it is still a little tough, return to the oven for a further 30 minutes.

For the lemony kale, steam the kale for 2 minutes until tender and bright green. Drain well and sprinkle over the lemon juice. Serve with the stew.

5 WAYS WITH *chicken breasts*

A healthy intake of protein is vital when your body is fighting cancer, and chicken is a great source of all the essential amino acids. Take a fresh, new look at chicken dishes to cook. Each of these suggestions serves 4.

Coconut and lime roasted chicken
Toss 4 chicken breasts in 120ml coconut milk, the grated zest and juice of 2 limes, 2 tsp grated ginger and 4 crushed garlic cloves. Roast at 200°C/Gas 6 for 20–25 minutes until cooked through. Serve with a salad of torn coriander, mint and basil leaves dressed with a squeeze of lime juice.

Pan-fried chicken with sage and Parma ham
Place 4 chicken breasts between 2 sheets of cling film and beat with a rolling pin to flatten to a 1cm thickness. Lay ½ slice of Parma ham on each chicken breast, top with a sage leaf and secure with a cocktail stick. Heat 2 tsp olive oil in a non-stick frying pan over a medium heat and fry the chicken breasts for 4–5 minutes on each side until cooked through. Season with black pepper and a squeeze of lemon juice. This is particularly good with the asparagus and bean salad on page 67.

Lemon, thyme and pine nut-crusted chicken
Beat 4 chicken breasts between 2 sheets of cling film with a rolling pin to flatten to a 1cm thickness. In a food processor, pulse the grated zest of 2 lemons, 2 crushed garlic cloves, 2 tbsp pine nuts, 2 tsp thyme leaves and 1 slice of wholemeal bread until the mixture resembles fine breadcrumbs. Stir through 2 tsp olive oil. Sprinkle over the chicken and bake at 200°C/Gas 6 for 20–25 minutes until cooked through. Serve with a tomato salad or the edamame salad on page 65.

Italian chicken grill
Place 4 chicken breasts in a large roasting tin with 400g cherry tomatoes, 2 roughly chopped aubergines, 2 roughly sliced courgettes, 4 crushed garlic cloves, 1 tbsp chopped oregano and 1 tbsp olive oil. Give it a good stir, season with pepper and roast at 200°C/Gas 6 for 25–30 minutes until the chicken is cooked through. Serve with a drizzle of balsamic vinegar and a scattering of basil.

Maple-glazed chicken and spring onion skewers
Cut 4 chicken breasts into bite-sized pieces and toss in a bowl with 4 tsp maple syrup, 1 tsp low-salt soy sauce and the juice of 1 lime. Marinate in the fridge for an hour. Cut 8 spring onions into 2cm lengths and thread onto skewers, alternating with the chicken. Grill for 10–12 minutes, turning frequently, until the chicken is cooked through and golden. Serve with soba noodles and a salad.

Vegetarian

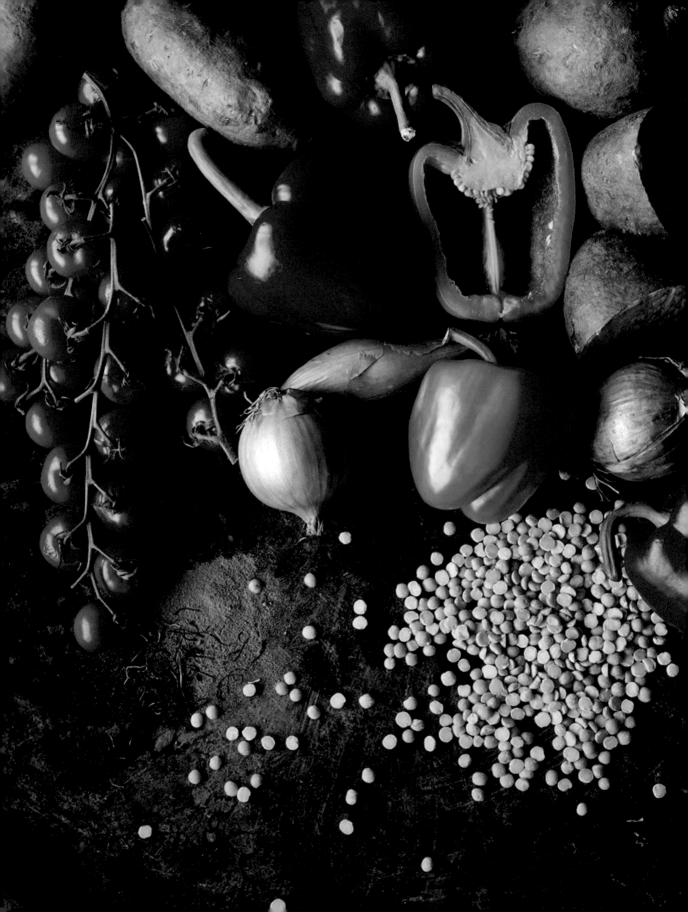

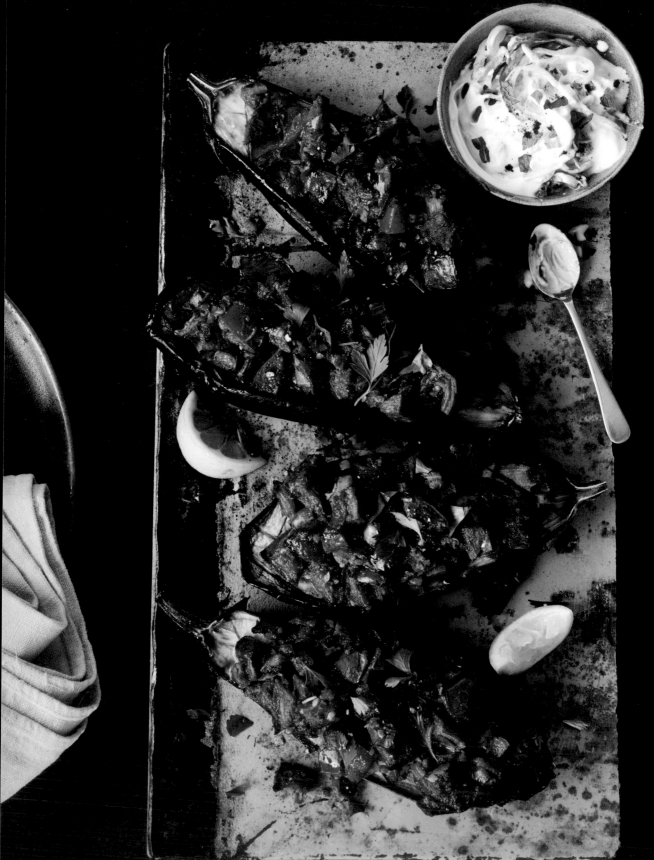

Imam bayildi with tzatziki and spelt flatbreads

Serves 4

For the aubergines

4 medium aubergines

3 tsp olive oil

1 large onion, peeled and chopped

3 garlic cloves, peeled and crushed

½ tsp ground cinnamon

1 tsp ground cumin

1 tbsp tomato purée

6 large tomatoes, roughly chopped

1 tsp maple syrup

Juice of 1 lemon

A small handful of parsley, roughly chopped

Freshly ground black pepper

For the tzatziki

½ cucumber, peeled, deseeded and grated

75g low-fat Greek yogurt

1 small garlic clove, peeled and crushed

A squeeze of lemon juice, to taste

1 tbsp finely chopped mint

A pinch of paprika, to serve

For the spelt flatbreads

250g wholemeal spelt flour, plus extra to dust

½ tsp dried oregano

A pinch of salt

1 tbsp baking powder

120–150ml warm water

2 tsp olive oil

This classic Turkish dish is warmed with cinnamon and cumin but you can omit these spices if you prefer – it will still be very tasty.

Preheat the oven to 180°C/Gas 4.

Halve the aubergines lengthways and score the flesh in a crisscross pattern. Brush with 1 tsp of the olive oil, transfer to a baking sheet and roast for 20 minutes, until tinged with brown at the edges.

Meanwhile, heat the remaining olive oil in a frying pan over a medium heat. Add the onion and fry gently for 5 minutes until softened. Add the garlic, cinnamon and cumin and fry for a further minute, until fragrant. Stir in the tomato purée, chopped tomatoes and maple syrup and remove from the heat.

Spoon the sauce on top of the aubergines and return to the oven for a further 20 minutes until the aubergines are soft and the sauce has reduced. Season with pepper to taste.

Meanwhile, for the tzatziki, put the grated cucumber in a clean tea towel and squeeze out the excess liquid, then transfer to a bowl and stir in the yogurt, garlic, lemon juice, mint and a little black pepper. Taste for seasoning and set aside.

For the flatbreads, sift the flour, oregano, salt and baking powder into a large bowl and make a well in the centre. Pour in 120ml warm water and the olive oil and quickly mix to a dough – if it's a bit dry, add a little more water.

Divide the dough into 8 pieces and roll each out on a lightly floured surface until about 5mm thick. Heat a large frying pan over a high heat and dry-fry the flatbreads for 1–2 minutes on each side until slightly risen and charred.

Sprinkle the baked aubergines with the lemon juice and parsley. Sprinkle the tzatziki with a little paprika. Serve the aubergines with the tzatziki and a flatbread or two. Although delicious hot, this dish is traditionally eaten cold, so save any leftovers for lunch the following day.

Ginger tempeh skewers with soba noodle salad

Serves 4

225g packet tempeh

2 tsp rice vinegar

2 tsp sesame oil

2 tsp clear honey

4 tsp low-salt soy sauce

2.5cm piece of fresh ginger, peeled and grated

2 small courgettes, each cut into 8 slices

8 shiitake mushrooms, halved

160g soba noodles

4 spring onions, finely sliced

100g radishes (large and/or small, finely sliced

100g sugar snap peas, halved

Juice of 1 lime

Tempeh, made from fermented and compressed soya beans, is like tofu's bigger and stronger cousin. It is delicious marinated in a honey and ginger dressing, then grilled with courgettes and mushrooms and served with a simple soba noodle and Asian vegetable salad.

Cut the tempeh into 16 equal-sized pieces. For the marinade, put the rice vinegar, sesame oil, honey, soy sauce and ginger into a ziplock bag and shake to combine. Add the tempeh, seal the bag and turn a few times to coat the tempeh in the marinade. Leave in the fridge for an hour.

While the tempeh is marinating, soak 8 wooden skewers in warm water (to prevent them catching and burning under the grill).

Preheat the grill to high. Remove the tempeh pieces from the marinade, reserving the marinade, and thread onto the wooden skewers, alternating with the courgette slices and mushrooms so that each skewer has 2 pieces of each.

Brush the tempeh skewers with a little of the marinade and grill for 5 minutes each side until golden and sticky.

Meanwhile, bring a pan of water to the boil. Add the soba noodles, give them a stir to stop them sticking together, and simmer for 6 minutes or according to the packet instructions. Drain and rinse under cold water to refresh. Drain well.

Toss the noodles in the reserved marinade and add the spring onions, radishes, sugar snaps and lime juice. Serve the tempeh skewers with the noodle salad.

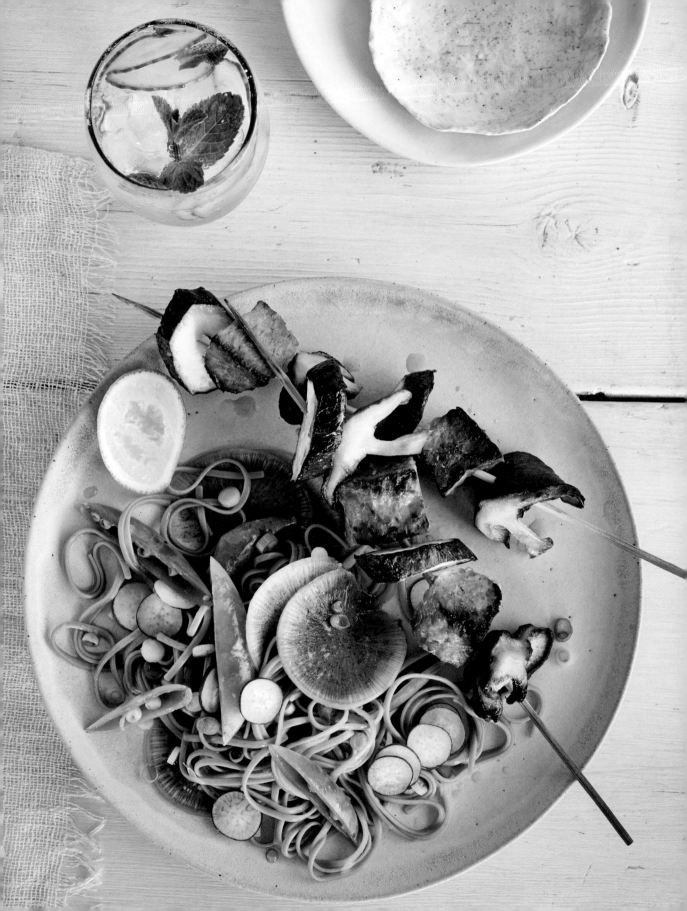

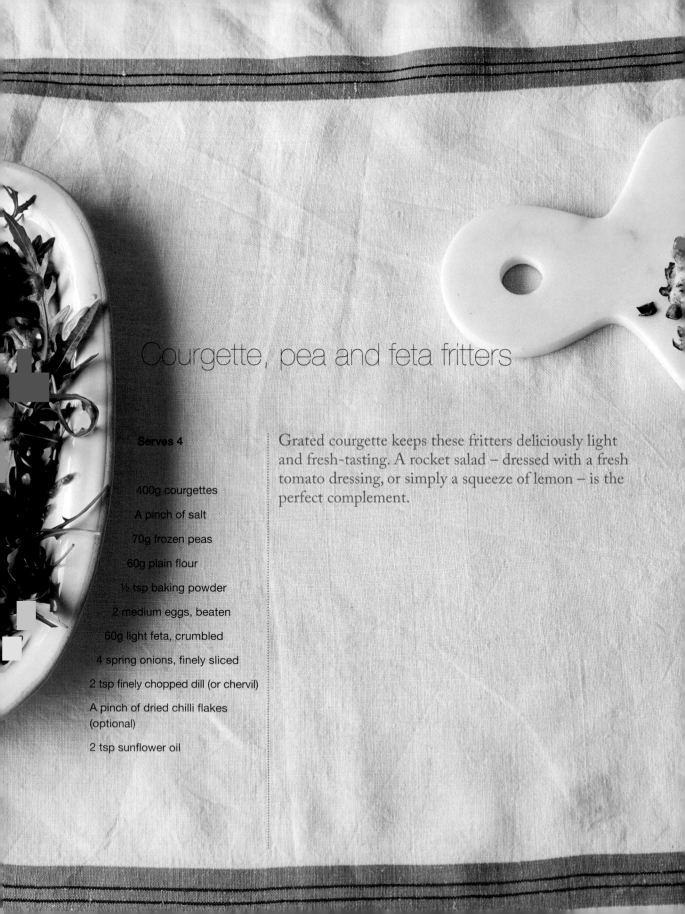

Courgette, pea and feta fritters

Serves 4

400g courgettes

A pinch of salt

70g frozen peas

60g plain flour

½ tsp baking powder

2 medium eggs, beaten

60g light feta, crumbled

4 spring onions, finely sliced

2 tsp finely chopped dill (or chervil)

A pinch of dried chilli flakes
(optional)

2 tsp sunflower oil

Grated courgette keeps these fritters deliciously light and fresh-tasting. A rocket salad – dressed with a fresh tomato dressing, or simply a squeeze of lemon – is the perfect complement.

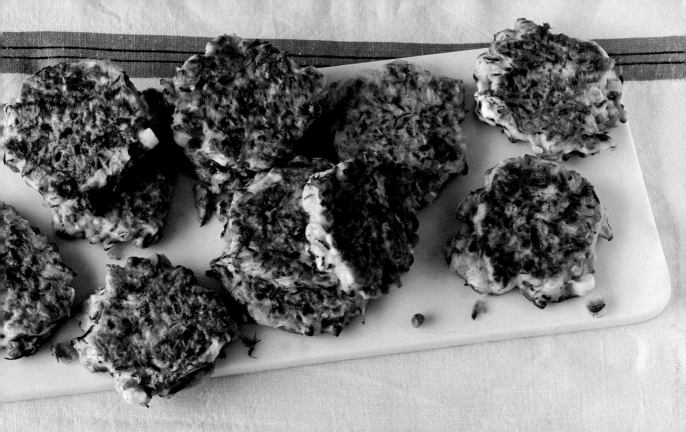

To serve

100g rocket leaves

1 quantity Fresh tomato and herb dressing (page 81), optional

1 lemon

Coarsely grate the courgettes and place in a colander set over a bowl. Sprinkle with a good pinch of salt, toss well and press down hard on the courgette several times. Set aside to drain for about 30 minutes, then squeeze out the excess water until the courgette is fairly dry (this will also exude the salt).

Meanwhile, tip the peas into a small, heatproof bowl. Just cover with boiling water and leave for 1 minute, then drain and set aside.

Sift the flour and baking powder into a large bowl and make a well in the centre. Add the eggs to the well and beat, gradually drawing in the flour, to create a smooth batter. Stir in the courgettes, peas, feta, spring onions, dill and chilli flakes, if using.

Heat a large, non-stick frying pan over a medium-high heat and add 1 tsp of the oil. Place 3 or 4 heaped spoonfuls of the courgette mixture in the pan, spacing them a little apart, and flatten slightly with the back of the spoon. Fry for 2 minutes on each side, until golden and crisp, then transfer to a plate lined with kitchen paper and keep warm. Repeat with the remaining mixture, adding more oil to the pan and adjusting the heat as necessary.

Dress the rocket leaves with the tomato dressing and serve with the lemon, cut into wedges. Alternatively, just sprinkle the rocket leaves with lemon juice and serve.

Sweet potato and sugar snap curry with fried cauliflower 'rice'

Serves 4

1 lemongrass stalk

2 tsp vegetable oil

3 tbsp red Thai curry paste

2 garlic cloves, peeled and crushed

2.5cm piece of fresh ginger, peeled and grated

300ml carrot juice or low-salt vegetable stock

400ml can low-fat coconut milk

600g sweet potatoes, peeled and cut into bite-sized chunks

1 medium cauliflower

150g cherry tomatoes, halved

1 yellow pepper, cored, deseeded and roughly chopped

200g sugar snap peas

Finely grated zest and juice of 1 lime

A handful of coriander leaves, roughly chopped

This mild Thai-style curry uses carrot juice rather than stock, which lends a touch of sweetness and flavour.

Bruise the lemongrass stalk with the back of a knife, remove the coarse outer layers and finely slice the tender inner part. Heat 1 tsp of the oil in a large wok over a medium heat. Add the curry paste, garlic, ginger and lemongrass and fry for 2 minutes until fragrant and golden.

Pour in the carrot juice or stock and the coconut milk and stir to combine. Bring to the boil, then add the sweet potatoes. Lower the heat slightly and simmer for 20 minutes until the potatoes have softened.

Meanwhile, cut the cauliflower into florets and pulse in a food processor (or coarsely grate) until it resembles grains of rice. Set aside.

Add the cherry tomatoes and yellow pepper to the curry and simmer for 3 minutes, then add the sugar snaps and cook for a further 2 minutes.

While the vegetables are cooking, heat the remaining oil in a large frying pan over a medium heat and add the cauliflower 'rice'. Fry for 5 minutes until it is tender and beginning to turn golden. Scatter over the lime zest.

Sprinkle the lime juice and coriander over the curry and serve with the fried cauliflower 'rice'.

Split pea and coconut dhal with carrot and coriander salad

Serves 4

For the dhal

250g yellow split peas (chana dhal), rinsed well

2 tsp vegetable oil

1 onion, peeled and finely chopped

3 garlic cloves, peeled and crushed

2.5cm piece of fresh ginger, peeled and grated

1 green chilli, deseeded for less heat (if preferred) and finely chopped

2 tsp ground cumin

1 tsp ground coriander

1 tsp ground turmeric

4 large tomatoes, roughly chopped

200ml low-fat coconut milk

Freshly ground black pepper

For the salad

4 medium carrots

A handful of coriander leaves, roughly chopped

Juice of 1 lime

Rich, creamy and aromatic, dhal is the ultimate healthy comfort food. Pairing it with a carrot and coriander salad gives you a vibrant, fresh-tasting meal that is also deeply satisfying.

In a medium pan, bring about 1 litre of water to the boil and stir in the split peas. Skim off any scum from the surface and put the lid on the pan. Simmer over a medium heat for 30 minutes, adding more water if necessary, until the peas are just tender. Remove from the heat and leave to cool.

Meanwhile, heat the oil in a large saucepan over a medium-low heat. Add the onion and fry gently for 5 minutes until softened. Add the garlic, ginger, chilli, cumin, coriander and turmeric and fry for 2 minutes, stirring regularly, until fragrant.

Add the tomatoes and coconut milk and simmer for 10–15 minutes, until thickened and reduced slightly.

Meanwhile for the salad, using a vegetable peeler, cut the carrots lengthways into long ribbons and place in a bowl. Add the coriander and lime juice and toss to combine.

Spoon the cooked lentils into the sauce, stir to combine and season with black pepper to taste. Bring to the boil, stirring, then remove from the heat.

Serve the dhal with the carrot and coriander salad alongside.

Saffron and spring vegetable quinoa pilaf

Serves 4

2 tsp olive oil

1 small red onion, peeled and finely chopped

2 leeks, well washed and finely sliced

2 garlic cloves, peeled and crushed

½ tsp ground turmeric

200g quinoa

A pinch of saffron strands

750ml–1 litre hot vegetable stock

200g asparagus spears

200g broccoli, cut into florets

200g petits pois

30g dried apricots, roughly chopped

Finely grated zest and juice of ½ lemon

2 tbsp mint leaves, roughly chopped

1 tbsp roughly chopped chives

2 tbsp parsley leaves, chopped

In this pilaf, sweet, tender vegetables and quinoa are warmed by saffron and turmeric and pepped up with fresh herbs and lemon – perfectly capturing the flavours of spring.

Heat the olive oil in a large sauté pan over a medium-low heat. Add the onion and leeks and fry gently for about 5 minutes until softened. Add the garlic and turmeric and continue to fry for a further 2 minutes, until fragrant.

Add the quinoa to the pan and stir for about a minute to allow the grains to toast. Crumble the saffron into the stock and pour 750ml stock into the pan. Bring back to a simmer, then cover and leave to steam for 8 minutes, until the grains are almost tender and the majority of the stock has been absorbed.

Meanwhile, snap off the woody ends of the asparagus and cut the spears into roughly 3cm lengths. Add to the pan with the broccoli and stir through the quinoa. If the mixture looks at all dry, pour in a little more stock.

Cover and cook gently for a further 4 minutes until the vegetables are tender. Add the peas, stir to distribute and then remove from the heat. Add a little more stock to moisten if necessary.

Stir through the dried apricots, lemon zest and juice and the chopped herbs and serve immediately.

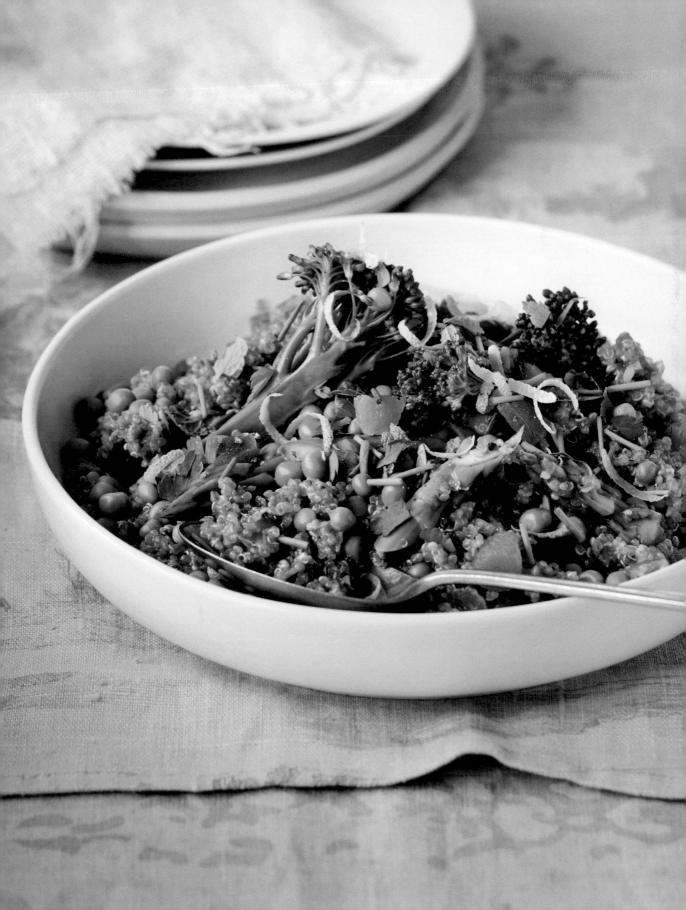

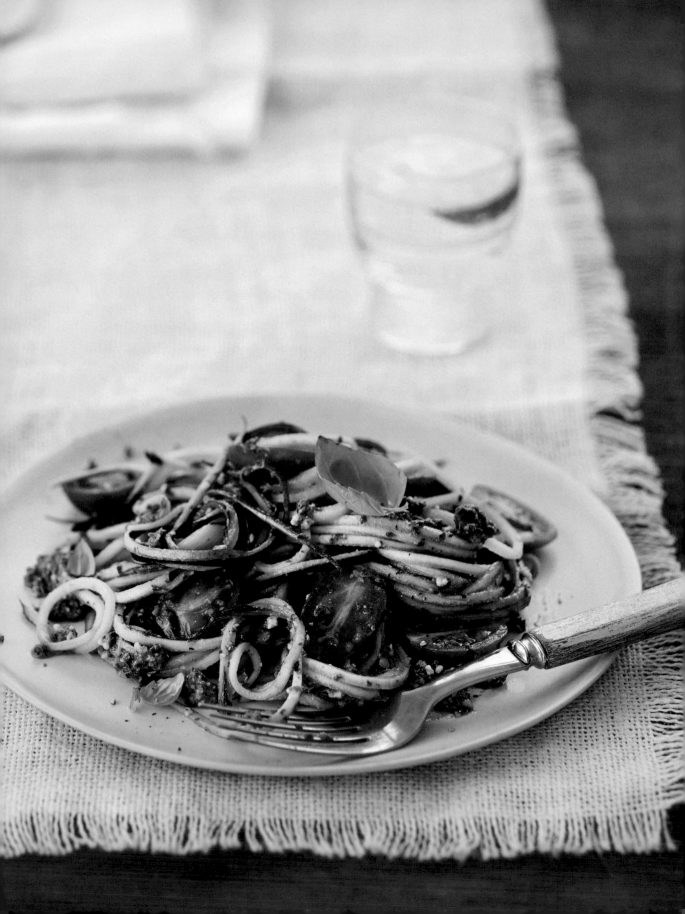

Courgette 'pasta' with kale, basil and sun-dried tomato pesto

Serves 4

4 medium courgettes

40g raw almonds

40g kale, roughly chopped, tough stalks discarded

40g basil leaves, plus a few extra to serve

8 sun-dried tomatoes (not in oil), rehydrated in warm water for 10 minutes

Juice of 1 lemon

1 tbsp olive oil

100g baby plum tomatoes, halved

Freshly ground black pepper

'Courgetti', or raw courgette shredded into strands like spaghetti, is exceptionally good – especially when it is teamed with a punchy basil pesto. This nutrient-packed raw veg dish is just as flavoursome as its more familiar pasta-based alternative.

To make the 'pasta', shred the courgettes using a julienne peeler to create strands, or a regular vegetable peeler to form ribbons. Set aside in a large bowl.

Put the almonds in a food processor and pulse until they have broken up into smaller pieces. Add the kale, basil, drained tomatoes and lemon juice and pulse again to create a thick paste. Add the olive oil and blend again. If the mixture is a little thick, add 1 tbsp or so of cold water.

Stir the pesto through the courgette 'pasta' with the baby plum tomatoes and serve scattered with plenty of black pepper and a few extra basil leaves.

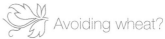 Avoiding wheat?

Try this appealing wheat-free 'pasta' dish that's packed with flavour. For anyone with coeliac disease, wheat allergy or gluten sensitivity, food choices are limited, unless you pay over the odds for 'gluten-free' alternatives, which are typically higher in fat due to product flavour modifications used to compensate for the removal of gluten. Gluten is found in so many products – bread, cereals, pasta, pizza and soy sauce, to name but a few. The innovative use of vegetables can help to make a gluten-free diet that much more interesting.

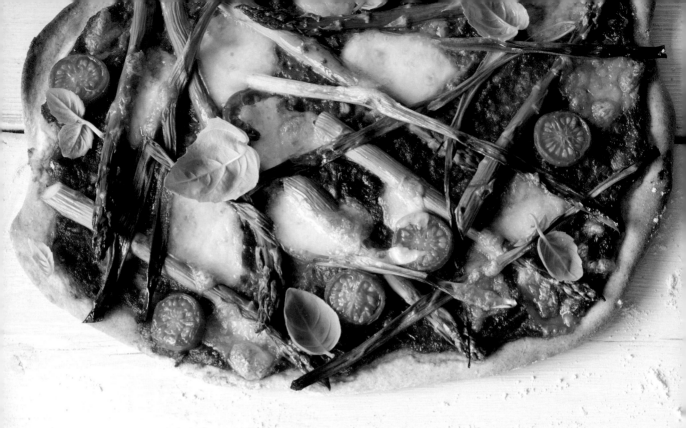

Speedy spelt pizzas

Makes 2 large pizzas (to serve 2–4, depending on appetite)

Ideal for a quick midweek supper, these homemade pizzas can be prepared and ready to eat in a matter of minutes. Spelt flour creates a delicious, nutty base and the dough is leavened with baking powder rather than yeast for a fast rise.

For the tomato sauce

1 tsp olive oil
2 shallots, peeled and finely chopped

2 garlic cloves, peeled and crushed

300ml passata

2 tbsp tomato purée

1 tsp dried oregano

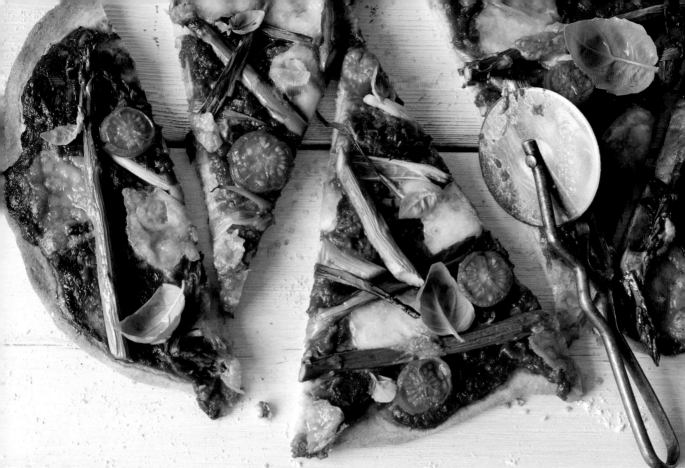

For the base

250g wholemeal spelt flour, plus extra to dust

1 tbsp baking powder

A pinch of salt

2 tsp olive oil

120–150ml warm water

For the topping

200g asparagus spears

6 spring onions, halved lengthways

100g cherry tomatoes, halved

120g mozzarella, torn into small pieces

A handful of basil leaves

Preheat the oven to 220°C/Gas 7.

To make the tomato sauce, heat the olive oil in a large frying pan and add the shallots. Fry for 2–3 minutes, until softened, then add the garlic and fry for a further minute until fragrant and golden. Stir in the passata, tomato purée and oregano and bring back to the boil. Simmer for about 5 minutes until the sauce is of a thick, spreadable consistency. Set aside to cool.

To make the pizza bases, sift the spelt flour, baking powder and salt into a large bowl and make a well in the centre. Pour the olive oil and 120ml water into the well and quickly mix to make a fairly stiff dough; if it is a little too dry, add an extra 1–2 tbsp water. Divide the dough in half.

Lightly flour 2 baking sheets, about 35 x 25cm. Place one piece of dough in the centre of one of the baking sheets and roll out until the dough reaches the edges of the sheet to form a large, rectangular base. Repeat with the other portion of dough.

Snap off the woody ends of the asparagus and cut the spears in half. Spread the tomato sauce over each pizza base, leaving a 1cm clear margin around the edges. Scatter the spring onions, asparagus, tomatoes and mozzarella over the pizzas and bake in the oven for 8–10 minutes until the base is crisp and puffed up and the cheese is melted. Serve immediately, scattered with the basil leaves.

Poached egg on za'atar kale with almond houmous

Serves 2

For the almond houmous

75g raw almonds, soaked in water overnight in the fridge

1 tbsp tahini

1 tsp olive oil

1 small garlic clove, peeled

¼ tsp ground cumin

Juice of 1 lemon

2–4 tbsp water

For the eggs

2 very fresh large eggs, chilled

For the kale

¼ tsp dried thyme

½ tsp ground sumac

1 tsp sesame seeds

200g kale, roughly chopped, tough stalks discarded

4 sun-dried tomatoes (not in oil), rehydrated in warm water for 10 minutes, drained and finely chopped

A squeeze of lemon juice

Freshly ground black pepper

This Middle Eastern inspired dish makes a satisfying and flavoursome meal at any time of day. The houmous can be prepared in advance and kept in the fridge for up to 3 days – you might like to double the quantity and enjoy the rest as a snack.

To make the houmous, drain the soaked almonds and place in a food processor. Add the tahini, olive oil, garlic and cumin and process to a rough paste. Add half of the lemon juice and 2 tbsp water and blitz again until smooth. Taste the houmous and add a little more lemon juice if required. If the houmous is still too thick, add up to another 2 tbsp water to let it down. Scoop into a bowl, cover and refrigerate until ready to serve.

To poach the eggs, fill a non-stick frying pan with a 4cm depth of water and bring to a simmer. Crack the eggs into small bowls or ramekins and tip them, one at a time, into the water. Allow to simmer gently for 3 minutes, then remove with a slotted spoon and drain on kitchen paper.

Meanwhile, heat a large dry frying pan over a medium heat and add the dried thyme, sumac and sesame seeds. Toast until golden and fragrant – about 1 minute. Add the kale with a splash of water and cook for 1 minute, until the kale has wilted. Remove from the heat and stir in the chopped sun-dried tomatoes and lemon juice.

Serve each portion of kale topped with a poached egg and a good grinding of black pepper, with a dollop of houmous on the side.

Roasted cauliflower with almonds

Serves 4

1 large cauliflower

2 tsp olive oil

2 garlic cloves, peeled and crushed

1 tsp ground cumin

1 tsp smoked paprika

40g raw almonds, roughly chopped

Juice of 1 lime

A small handful of coriander leaves, roughly chopped

If you haven't roasted cauliflower before, prepare for a revelation. A golden char on the edge of a floret brings out the sweet nuttiness of the vegetable, while the aromatics and almonds in this dish add a warming wholesomeness. This dish is great as a side but it can be a complete meal with the addition of herby quinoa and steamed greens, or a simple salad.

Preheat the oven to 200°C/Gas 6.

Halve the cauliflower vertically and cut each half into 1cm thick slices. Pile into a large bowl and add the olive oil, garlic, cumin and smoked paprika. Give it a good stir, so the cauliflower slices are evenly coated.

Transfer the cauliflower to a baking sheet or roasting tin, placing the slices in a single layer, and roast for 10 minutes.

Remove from the oven, turn the cauliflower pieces over and scatter over the chopped almonds. Roast for a further 10 minutes until the cauliflower is charred at the edges and tender. Sprinkle with the lime juice and coriander and serve.

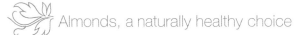 Almonds, a naturally healthy choice

Nuts and seeds provide a powerful complex of phytonutrients, unsaturated fats, soluble fibre and antioxidant vitamins, shown to reduce blood glucose and lower cholesterol levels. Although high-energy ingredients, they are generally consumed in modest amounts and not typically associated with weight gain. As with most foods, natural (unroasted and unsalted) almonds – eaten with their skins intact – provide the greatest benefits as many of the nutrients are concentrated in, or just beneath, the skin.

Okra, aubergine and tomato stir-fry

Serves 4

2 medium aubergines

250g okra

2 tsp olive oil

2 fat garlic cloves, peeled and finely sliced

1½ tbsp tomato purée

200g cherry tomatoes, halved

3 tsp low-salt soy sauce

80g baby spinach leaves

Lime wedges, to serve

Okra and aubergine are stir-fried with tomatoes and soy until crisp and pillowy – to create a tempting dish with a rich, savoury umami flavour. Enjoy as a side dish or as a meal in itself with steamed brown rice.

Halve the aubergines lengthways, then cut them across into 1cm thick slices. Trim the stalk ends of the okra, then cut the pods in half lengthways.

Heat half of the olive oil in a large, non-stick frying pan or wok over a medium-high heat. When the oil is hot, add the aubergine slices and fry for 1–2 minutes on each side, until well browned (you may have to do this in 2 batches to avoid overcrowding the pan). Remove from the pan and set aside.

Fry the okra in the same way, in the remaining oil, for 1–2 minutes each side. Add the garlic to the pan and fry for a further minute.

Return the aubergine to the pan and add the tomato purée, cherry tomatoes and soy sauce. Stir-fry for 1–2 minutes until the tomatoes begin to break down. Now add the spinach and stir briefly, then remove from the heat.

Divide the stir-fry between warmed bowls and serve straight away, with lime wedges.

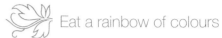 Eat a rainbow of colours

Advice suggests that at least half of every plate we eat should comprise fruit and/or vegetables. Being reactive to the plethora of colours that these ingredients offer will not only provide diversity within the diet, but also an extensive range of nutrients – to create an appetising, nutritious meal.

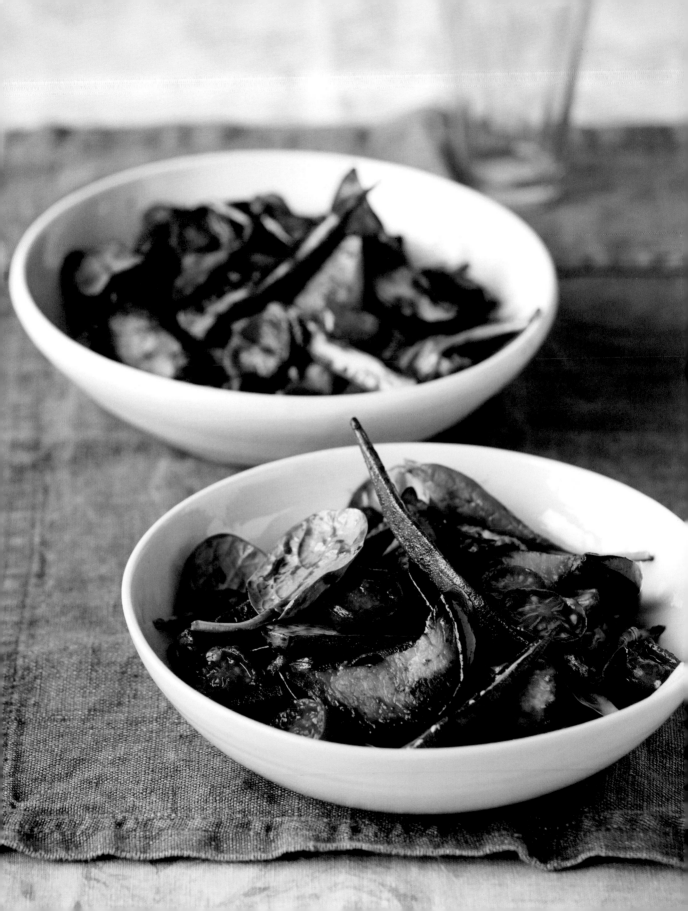

Braised chicory and fennel

Serves 4

4 chicory bulbs

2 small fennel bulbs

2 tsp olive oil

2 garlic cloves, peeled and crushed

150ml low-salt chicken stock

2 tsp thyme leaves, roughly chopped

Juice of ½ lemon

2 tbsp chopped parsley

Freshly ground black pepper

This simple and delicate dish makes for a wonderful vegetarian side. To enjoy as a main dish, serve with a robust salad, such as the Asparagus and white bean salad on page 67.

Peel away any tired-looking outer leaves from the chicory and cut in half lengthways. Remove any tough outer layer from the fennel and roughly cut into wedges lengthways.

Heat the olive oil in a sauté pan or large frying pan over a medium heat. Add the fennel and chicory and fry for 1–2 minutes on each side, until golden (you may need to do this in 2 batches to avoid overcrowding the pan). Add the garlic and fry gently for a further minute, until fragrant and softened.

Return all the fennel and chicory to the pan (if browned in batches) and pour over the stock. Scatter over the thyme and season with a little black pepper. Bring to a simmer, lower the heat and braise gently, stirring gently occasionally, for 20–25 minutes until the veg are meltingly soft at the edges but still firm to the bite within.

Sprinkle with the lemon juice, scatter over the chopped parsley and serve immediately.

5 WAYS WITH *leafy greens*

Consuming more of these vibrant, low-calorie vegetables can reduce the risk of developing stomach, breast and skin cancers, while also benefiting your cardiovascular and bone health. Beyond steamed spinach and boiled cabbage, there are so many more interesting ways to enjoy them. Here are five targeted recipes to get you started...

Japanese Swiss chard

Roughly chop 200g Swiss chard, including the colourful stems. Boil for 3 minutes, drain and submerge in iced water. Drain again and toss with 3 tsp low-salt soy sauce. Crumble over a sheet of nori and serve as a snack or appetiser. 4–6 servings

Roasted kale with Parmesan

Roughly chop 200g kale, discarding the central stalks. Toss in 1 tsp olive oil and 20g freshly grated Parmesan and transfer to a baking sheet. Bake in the oven at 140°C/ Gas 1 for 20–25 minutes until crisp. 3–4 servings

Quick spring green soup

Bring 1 litre low-salt vegetable stock to the boil in a saucepan. Add 200g finely chopped spring greens, 100g frozen peas and 100g watercress and cook for 1 minute. Serve sprinkled with 20g grated Parmesan, a squeeze of lemon juice and black pepper. 4 servings

Spinach with garlic, lemon and walnuts

Heat 1 tsp olive oil in a large frying and add 2 crushed garlic cloves, the finely grated zest of 1 lemon and 20g finely chopped walnuts. Fry for 2 minutes, then add 200g baby leaf spinach and wilt for 1 minute before serving. 4 servings

Stir-fried Savoy cabbage with almonds

Heat 2 tsp olive oil in a large frying pan. When hot, add 1 tsp caraway seeds and a shredded small Savoy cabbage. Fry for 2 minutes, then add 3 tbsp water and steam-fry for a further 3–4 minutes, until tender. Serve sprinkled with 20g roughly chopped raw almonds. 4 servings

Desserts and Treats

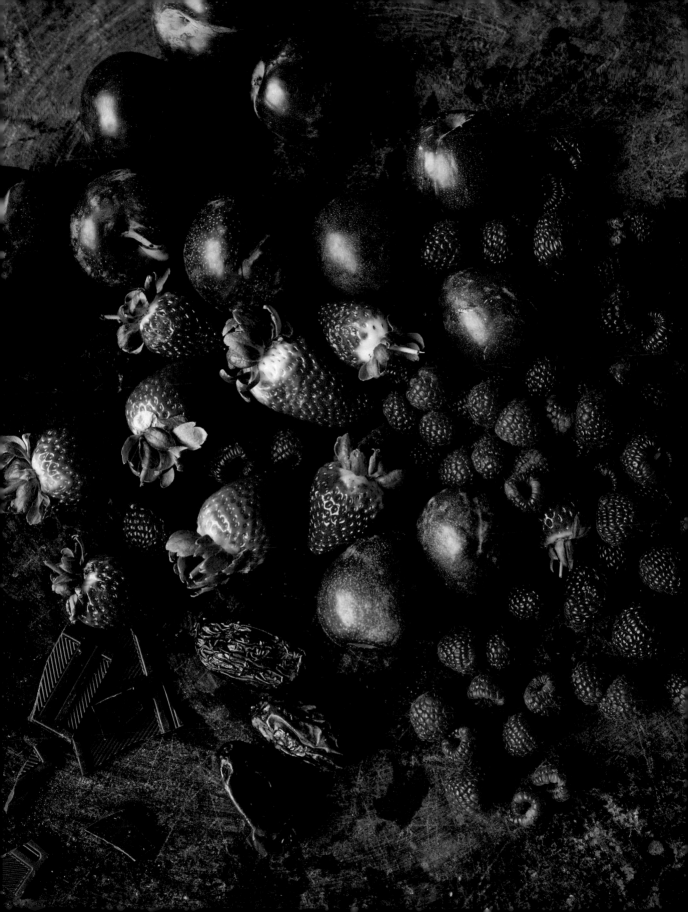

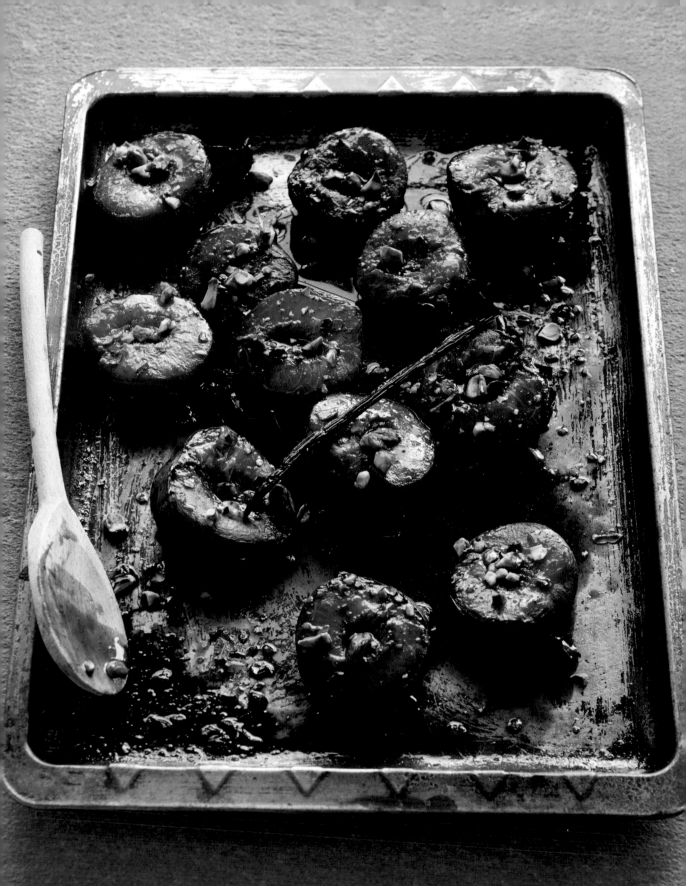

Roasted vanilla and orange plums with pistachios

Serves 4

6 ripe plums, halved and stoned

1 vanilla pod, halved lengthways and seeds scraped

Juice of 2 oranges

2 tsp maple syrup

3 tbsp water

30g pistachio nuts, roughly chopped

Roasting plums brings out their natural syrupy sweetness. Here orange juice and vanilla form a delectable fragrant syrup that enhances the flavour of the fruit, while a topping of chopped pistachios provides a contrasting crunch.

Preheat the oven to 180°C/Gas 4.

Place the plums, cut side up, in a baking dish large enough to fit them in one layer.

Stir the vanilla seeds into the orange juice and combine with the maple syrup and water.

Pour the juice mix over the plums, top with the vanilla pod and sprinkle over the pistachios. Bake in the oven for 25–30 minutes, until the plums are tender and syrupy. Serve warm, with a dollop of natural yogurt.

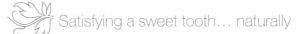 Satisfying a sweet tooth… naturally

Ripe fruits are naturally sweet and contain a breadth of nutritive benefits, so from an evolutionary perspective we are programmed to enjoy – and gain from – them. Desserts that are naturally rich in nutrient-rich sweetness, which do not call for the addition of cream or a calorie-laden sauce, belong in a healthy diet.

Oaty pear and blackberry crumble

Serves 4–6

For the filling

800g ripe pears

400g blackberries

40g sultanas, very roughly chopped

Juice of ½ lemon

2 tsp maple syrup

For the topping

50g raw almonds

100g rolled oats

1 tsp ground cinnamon

2 tsp maple syrup

2 tsp sunflower oil

This lighter take on a comforting crumble tastes just as good as the original. Ripe pears and blackberries need the minimum of additional sweetness and the granola-like topping lends a welcome crunch.

Preheat the oven to 200°C/Gas 6.

For the filling, peel, core and roughly chop the pears and place them in a medium saucepan with the blackberries, sultanas, lemon juice and maple syrup. Cook over a medium-low heat, stirring occasionally, for 5 minutes until the fruit is beginning to soften.

Transfer the fruit to a fairly shallow 1.5 litre baking dish and set aside while you prepare the topping.

For the topping, tip the almonds into a food processor and pulse until broken up into small chunks. Add the oats, cinnamon, maple syrup and oil and pulse a few more times until the mixture forms small clumps.

Sprinkle the topping evenly over the fruit and bake in the oven for 20 minutes, until the topping is golden and the filling is bubbling around the edges. Check the crumble during cooking – if the top is golden before 20 minutes have elapsed, cover loosely with foil for the rest of the cooking time.

Serve warm, with a spoonful of yogurt or low-fat crème fraîche.

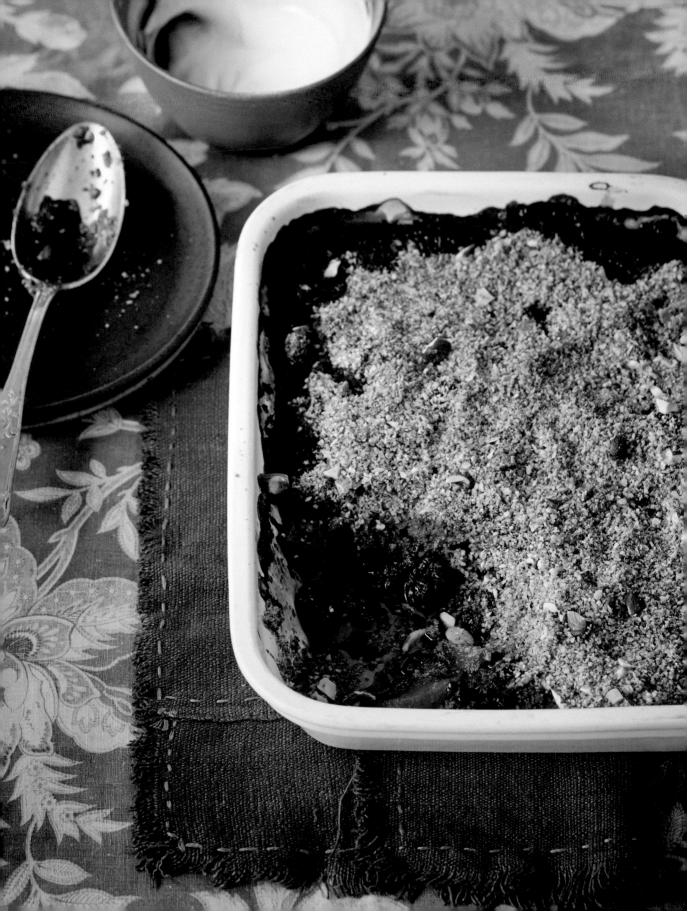

Baked stuffed apples
with cinnamon, dried figs and raisins

Serves 4

4 dessert apples, such as Braeburn

Juice of ½ lemon

50g raisins

50g dried figs, finely chopped

1 tsp maple syrup

1 tsp ground cinnamon

1 tsp butter

4 tbsp water

Enjoy this classic, autumnal dessert warm from the oven or cold with some natural yogurt. Easy to prepare, it's a lovely way to enjoy the apple harvest.

Preheat the oven to 180°C/Gas 4.

Using an apple corer, remove the cores from the apples and make a shallow cut around the circumference of each apple to stop the skin from splitting during cooking.

Stand the apples in a fairly deep baking dish and sprinkle over the lemon juice. Mix the raisins, figs, maple syrup and cinnamon together and spoon into the apple cavities, filling them to the top. Dot the top of each apple with butter and spoon the water into the bottom of the dish.

Cover the dish with foil and bake for 15 minutes, then remove the foil and bake for a further 10 minutes, until the apples have softened and the juices in the dish are syrupy. Serve warm, with a dollop of natural yogurt.

Pineapple and star anise carpaccio

Serves 4–6

2 tbsp maple syrup

1 star anise

Finely grated zest and juice of
1 lime

2 tbsp water

1 large ripe pineapple

2 tbsp mint leaves, roughly
chopped

This simple, vibrant dessert is just the thing to enjoy on a warm summer's eve. The aniseed fragrance from the star anise adds an enticing, warming spice to lively fresh pineapple.

Put the maple syrup, star anise, lime juice and water in a saucepan and place over a medium heat. Simmer for 5–10 minutes, until the mixture is of a light syrup consistency. Remove from the heat, discard the star anise and leave to cool.

Place the pineapple on a board and cut off the top and bottom. Slice down the sides of the pineapple to remove the skin and then prise out any brown 'eyes' that are left.

Turn the pineapple onto its side and slice as thinly as possible. Lay the slices out onto a serving dish and drizzle over the syrup. Sprinkle over the lime zest and mint leaves and serve.

If you are serving the carpaccio on a particularly hot day, lay the pineapple slices over a bed of crushed ice.

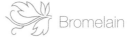 Bromelain

A natural enzyme found in pineapple, bromelain has been linked to the alleviation of symptoms associated with chemotherapy treatment, including inflammation and diarrhoea. As with many positive dietary cancer attestations, evidence is not yet conclusive, but inclusion of pineapple in the diet may alleviate joint and gastrointestinal upsets commonly experienced following chemotherapy treatment.

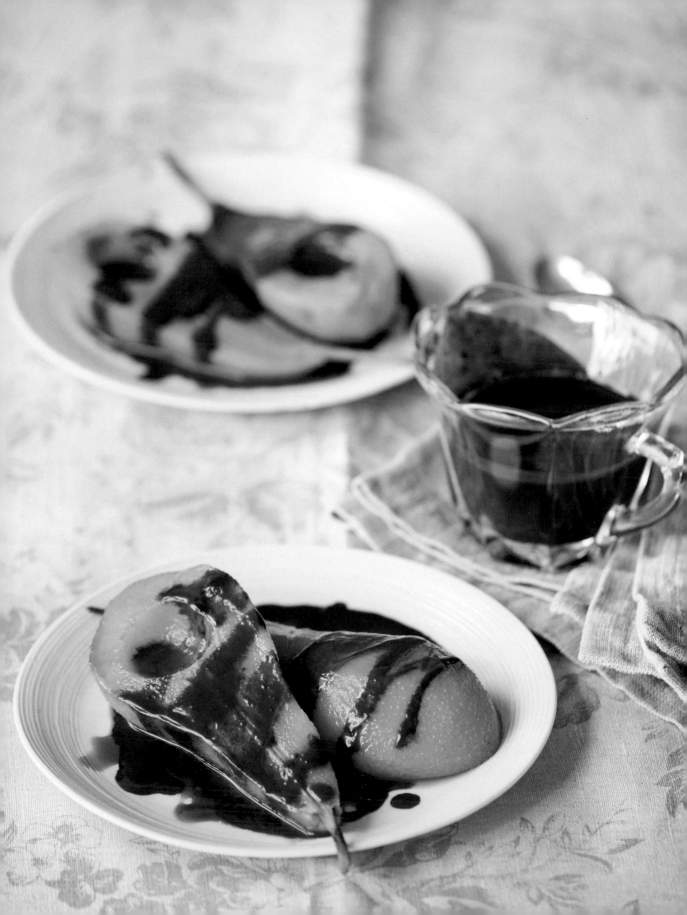

Earl Grey poached pears with warm chocolate sauce

Serves 4

3 Earl Grey tea bags

700ml boiling water

4 ripe pears

Juice of ½ lemon

2 tbsp clear honey

For the chocolate sauce

80g dark chocolate, minimum 70% cocoa solids

1 tsp vanilla extract

6 tbsp almond milk

Gently poaching pears with the subtle aromas of Earl Grey tea, instead of the usual alcohol and sugar-spiked liquor, renders them tender and fragrant. Cloaked in a warm chocolate sauce, they are wonderfully indulgent.

Immerse the tea bags in the boiling water and leave to infuse for 3 minutes, until fragrant. Strain the tea and set aside.

Carefully peel the pears. Using a teaspoon or melon baller, scoop out the core and cut out the woody base from each pear.

Stand the pears in a saucepan in which they fit quite snugly and sprinkle over the lemon juice and honey. Pour over the tea and place the pan over a medium-low heat. Bring to a simmer and cook gently, adjusting the heat if necessary, for 25 minutes until the pears are tender right through.

Lift out the pears with a slotted spoon, slice them in half and place in a bowl; keep warm.

Put the pan back over a high heat and let the liquor bubble for 5–10 minutes to reduce until syrupy. Set aside.

For the sauce, finely chop the chocolate and put into a heatproof bowl. Place over a pan of just-boiled water, ensuring that the base of the bowl is not in direct contact with the water. Allow the chocolate to melt, stirring occasionally. As soon as it has melted, remove the bowl from the pan. Stir in the vanilla extract and almond milk to make a thick sauce.

Serve 2 pear halves per person, drizzled with the reduced syrup and topped with the warm chocolate sauce.

Chocolate mousse with raspberries

Serves 4

100g dark chocolate, minimum 70% cocoa solids

100ml coconut milk

1 very ripe avocado

4 pitted Medjool dates, roughly chopped

1 tsp vanilla extract

200g raspberries

This luxurious dessert is the ultimate guilt-free indulgence for anybody wanting to eat more mindfully. The rich creaminess of avocado gives the mousse its silky texture whilst the fudgy sweetness of dates provides a foil for the tart raspberries.

Finely chop the chocolate and put into a heatproof bowl with the coconut milk. Place over a pan of just-boiled water, ensuring that the base of the bowl is not in direct contact with the water. Allow the chocolate to melt, stirring occasionally.

Once the chocolate has melted, remove the bowl from the pan and set aside to cool for 10 minutes.

Meanwhile, halve the avocado, remove the stone and scoop the flesh from the skin into a food processor. Add the dates and blend, scraping down the sides occasionally, until smooth and creamy; this should take 2–3 minutes.

Scrape the melted chocolate mixture into the food processor, add the vanilla extract and blend again for a couple of minutes, until smooth. Divide equally between 4 serving dishes. These mousses can be eaten straight away or chilled for a couple of hours before serving.

When ready to serve, roughly crush the raspberries in a bowl with the back of a fork. Serve the chocolate mousses topped with the crushed raspberries.

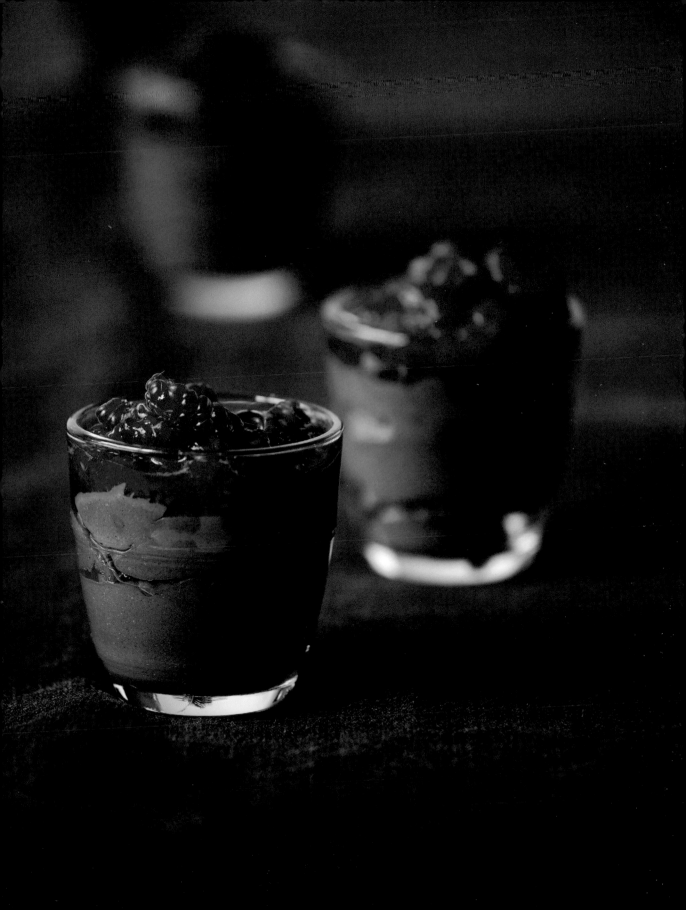

Banana and berry soft-serve ice

Serves 4

2 large, very ripe bananas

150g mixed berries, such as strawberries, raspberries and blueberries

To make this simple 'ice cream', all you need is the frozen fruit on standby and a food processor and you'll have a light, refreshing, sugar-free dessert in minutes.

Cut the bananas into 2cm thick slices and lay, slightly apart, on a baking sheet lined with baking parchment.

Hull the strawberries and place all the berries in a freezerproof container. Freeze the bananas and berries for at least 6 hours.

Tip the banana slices and berries into a food processor and process for 3–5 minutes, scraping down the sides of the bowl a few times, until the mixture is smooth and of a soft ice-cream consistency. Serve immediately.

Mango, coconut and lime ice cream

Serves 4

1 large ripe mango

200ml coconut milk

Finely grated zest and juice of
1 lime

This ice cream is made in moments from blended
frozen mango and coconut milk. The only sweetness
comes from the sticky, syrupy mango, so make sure you
use one that is ripe.

Peel the mango, cut the flesh from the stone, then cut into roughly
2cm chunks. Place in a freezerproof bowl and freeze for a minimum
of 6 hours.

Pour the coconut milk into ice-cube trays and freeze for 2–3 hours,
until firm and icy but not frozen solid.

Put the frozen mango, coconut milk cubes and the lime zest
and juice into a food processor and blend for about 5 minutes,
scraping down the sides every so often, until the mixture if of
a soft ice-cream consistency. Serve immediately.

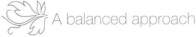 A balanced approach

Moderation and balance are key to any successful
healthy diet. Avoiding specific foods on the basis that
they are 'bad for us' can be counter-productive. Ice
creams and sorbets, for example, can form part of a
balanced meal if you make them yourself and typically
include fruit and other nutrient-rich ingredients. For
a contrast in texture, if required, serve them with fresh
fruit rather than dessert biscuits with a high fat content.

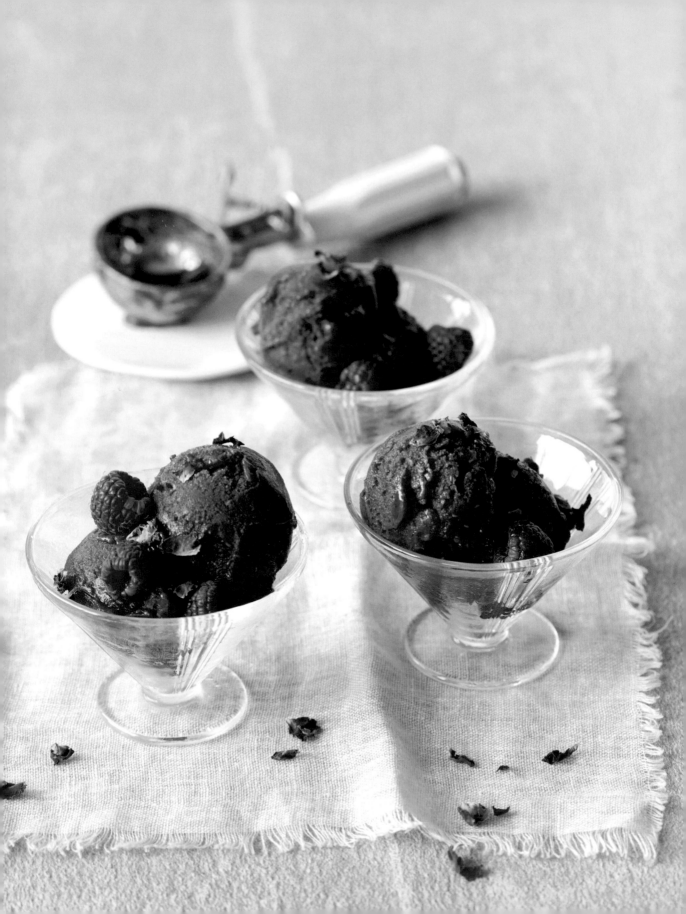

Berry and rosewater sorbet

Serves 4

250g strawberries, hulled

250g raspberries

¼ tsp rosewater

2 tsp maple syrup

2 tbsp water (if needed)

The subtle, floral aroma of rosewater complements the natural sweetness of berries in this refreshing sorbet.

Halve 150g of the strawberries and place these in a freezerproof container with all of the raspberries. Freeze for a minimum of 6 hours.

Once the fruit it completely frozen, transfer to a food processor and add the fresh strawberries, rosewater and maple syrup. Blend for about 5 minutes, scraping the sides down regularly, until you have a soft, spoonable sorbet.

If the mixture still seems very stiff after 5 minutes of blending, add 2 tbsp water and blend again. Serve immediately.

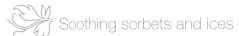 Soothing sorbets and ices

Sensitive gums and a sore mouth are a common consequence of cancer treatment and care must be taken to prevent localised infections, as your body has enough to cope with fighting cancer. Cold, smooth foods like ices and sorbets can provide a welcome relief from discomfort. Make your own soft ices and smoothies and use them as a means to introduce nutrient-rich fruits into your diet, remembering to avoid any ingredients known to irritate your mouth.

Pumpkin pie slices

Makes 16

For the filling

1 large butternut squash

100ml maple syrup

150ml coconut milk

3 large eggs, beaten

2 tsp vanilla extract

1 tsp ground cinnamon

¼ tsp ground nutmeg

For the base

100g pecan halves

75g ground almonds

25g rolled oats

2 Medjool dates, roughly chopped

1 large egg, beaten

This lovely traybake gives you all the warming flavours of a traditional pumpkin pie in a little slice. Once cooled, the slices can be kept in the fridge for 2–3 days.

Preheat the oven to 200°C/Gas 6.

Cut the squash in half, remove the seeds and wrap each half in foil. Place in a roasting tray and bake in the oven for 1–1½ hours until completely tender. Remove from the oven, open up the foil and set aside to cool.

Turn the oven down to 180°C/Gas 4. Lightly grease and line a 23cm square shallow baking tin with baking parchment.

While the squash is cooling, prepare the base. Tip the pecans into a food processor and blitz for 2–3 minutes, until the nuts start to clump together. Add the remaining ingredients and blend to a fairly sticky dough.

Using wet hands, press the dough onto the base of the prepared tin as evenly as you can. Bake in the oven for 8 minutes, until beginning to turn golden. Remove and set aside to cool while you prepare the filling.

Scoop the cooled flesh from the squash; you should have about 600g. Spoon into the cleaned food processor, add the rest of the filling ingredients and blend until smooth and creamy. Pass the mixture through a sieve and spread evenly over the base.

Bake in the oven for 25–30 minutes, until the filling is just set. Leave to cool and then chill to firm up before serving. Cut into 16 squares to serve.

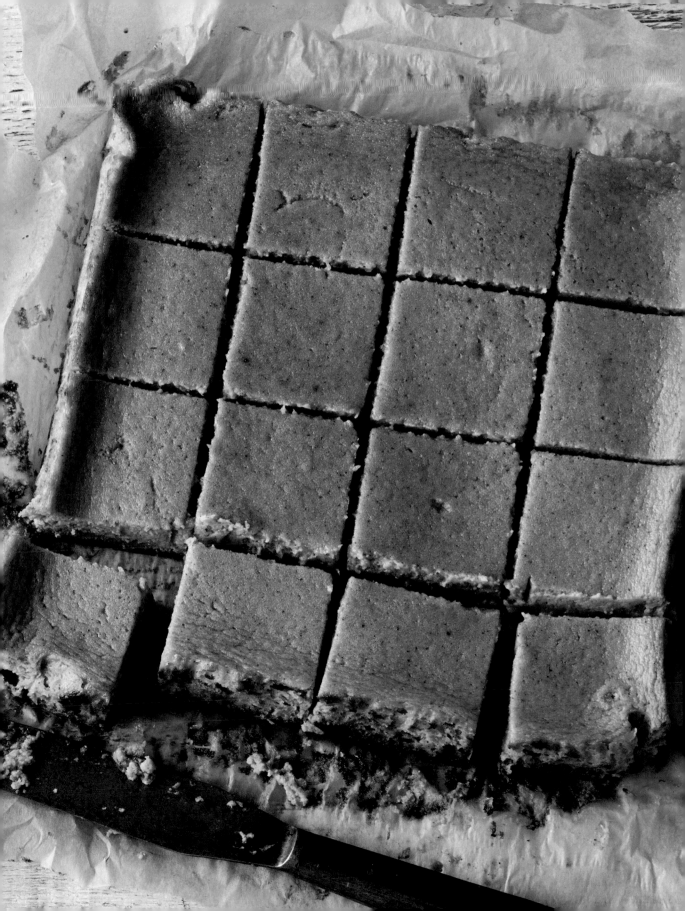

Apple, almond and cinnamon cake

Makes 12 slices

4 dessert apples

Juice of ½ lemon

100g sultanas, chopped
fairly finely

2 tbsp water

4 large egg whites

2 tbsp maple syrup

50g plain wholemeal flour

100g ground almonds

1 tsp ground cinnamon

1 tsp baking powder

2 tbsp sunflower oil

This delicate cake is made with a maple meringue to keep it light and fluffy. Wrapping the hot cake in a tea towel as it cools helps to retain the delicious moisture from the fruits.

Preheat the oven to 180°C/Gas 4. Lightly grease an 18cm springform cake tin and line with baking parchment.

Peel the apples and chop all but one into fairly small chunks. Quarter and core the other apple, then cut into fairly thin slices. Sprinkle all of the apple pieces with the lemon juice.

Put the chopped apples into a saucepan with the sultanas and water. Place over a medium-low heat and simmer gently for 10–15 minutes, stirring regularly, until the apples are fairly soft. Tip the mixture into a bowl and set aside to cool.

In a clean bowl, whisk the egg whites until they form stiff peaks. Trickle over the maple syrup and whisk again until stiff.

Sift the flour, ground almonds, cinnamon and baking powder together over the egg whites, tipping in any bran and almonds that remain in the sieve. Carefully fold the flour and almond mixture into the meringue with a spatula or large metal spoon until just combined. Finally, fold in the cooled fruit.

Spoon the mixture into the prepared tin and gently smooth the surface with a spatula. Arrange the apple slices on top of the cake in concentric circles. Bake in the oven for 30–35 minutes, until golden and a cocktail stick inserted into the centre of the cake comes out clean.

Leave the cake to cool in the tin for 10 minutes before turning out. Wrap the warm cake in a tea towel as it cools and serve warm or at room temperature. Once cooled, it will keep for 2–3 days stored in an airtight container.

5 WAYS WITH *dried fruit*

Changes in taste perception following breast cancer treatment can lead to avoidance of acidic fresh fruits. Dried fruits offer a compact, easily transportable alternative with a multitude of uses. They have a concentrated, positive nutrient profile – containing valuable micro-nutrients, phytochemicals and soluble fibre. Try these luscious suggestions to increase your intake.

Chocolate and date truffles
In a food processor, blitz 100g pitted Medjool dates with 75g desiccated coconut, 75g ground almonds, 4 tbsp cocoa powder and 1 tbsp melted coconut oil until the mixture forms a dough. Roll into 16 balls and store in the fridge for up to 4 days.

Healthy fruit bars
Line a 23cm square shallow baking tin with baking parchment. Blend 100g dried figs, 100g dried apricots, 1 tbsp melted coconut oil and 100g raw cashew nuts until smooth, and spread in the prepared tin. Place in the fridge for 2 hours to set, then slice into 16 bars.

Apricot paste
Put 200g organic (unsulphured) dried apricots in a bowl, pour on 300ml boiled water and leave to soak for 30 minutes, until plump. Blend until smooth and use to sweeten cakes, yogurt – even salad dressings.

Cranberry roasted veg
Roast carrots, parsnips and celeriac in a little olive oil and sprinkle with a spoonful of dried cranberries to serve.

Sticky prune porridge
Make porridge with 50g rolled oats and 250–300ml milk, and flavour with a pinch of ground cinnamon. Roughly chop 3 prunes and stir through the porridge to serve.

Drinks

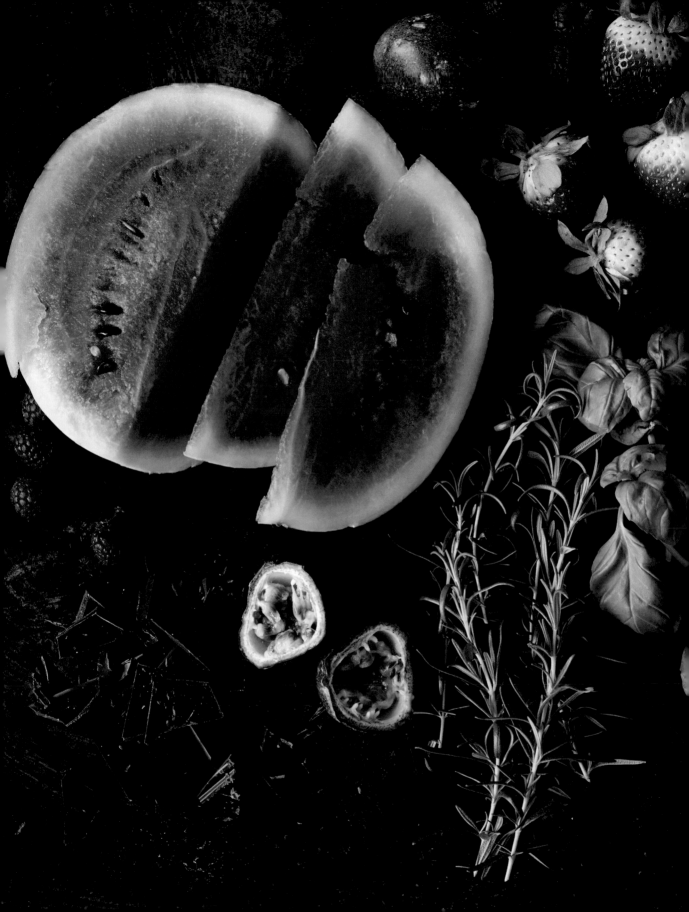

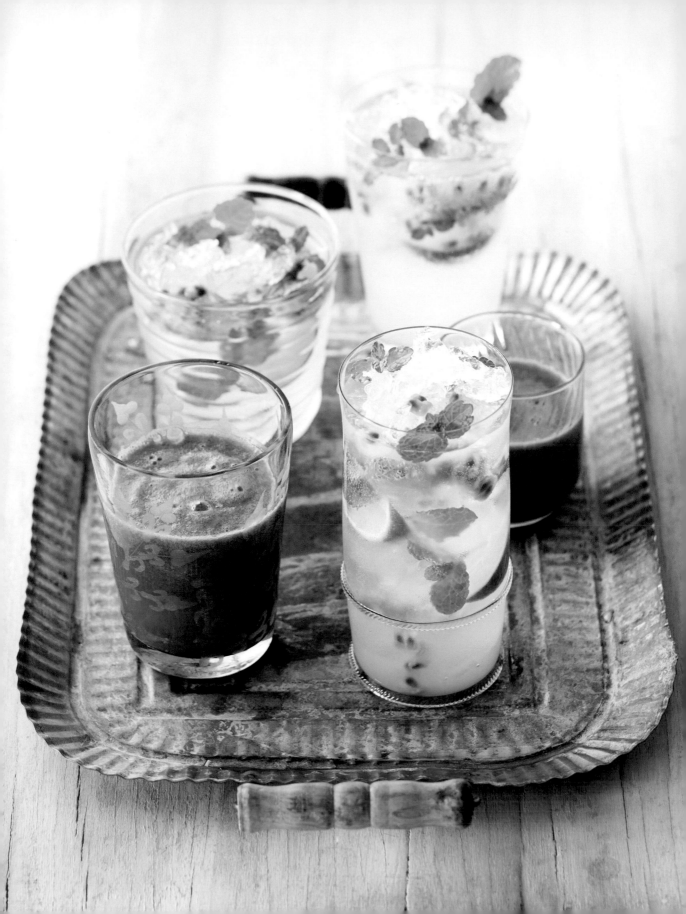

Passion fruit and mint cooler

Serves 2

1 passion fruit

½ lime, cut into wedges

2 tbsp mint leaves

Sparkling water, to top up

Crushed ice, to serve

This refreshing summer drink will be perfectly cooling on a hot summer's day.

Halve the passion fruit and scoop out the pulp and seeds with a teaspoon into a measuring jug. Add the lime wedges and mint leaves and lightly crush the ingredients together with a wooden spoon until juicy.

Half-fill two glasses with crushed ice and spoon over the crushed fruit and mint mix. Top up with sparking water, stir and serve.

Watermelon, ginger and lemon juice

Serves 4

750g watermelon flesh, cut into chunks

1cm piece of fresh ginger, peeled

Juice of 1 lemon

Ice cubes, to serve

The sweetness of watermelon is given an edge with spicy ginger and citrusy lemon.

Put the watermelon, ginger and lemon juice in a food processor and blitz thoroughly. There is no need to remove the watermelon pips first as blending will grind them down, but if you would prefer a velvety smooth result, strain the juice before serving over ice.

Lemongrass, ginger and lime infusion

Serves 2

1 lemongrass stalk

1cm piece of fresh ginger, peeled and sliced

½ lime, cut into wedges

600ml boiling water

This aromatic blend is a wonderfully cleansing drink to enjoy first thing in the morning.

Bruise the lemongrass stalk with the back of a knife and slice in half. Divide the lemongrass, ginger and lime between 2 large mugs and pour over the boiling water. Leave to infuse for 3–5 minutes before drinking.

Mayan almond hot chocolate

Serves 2

50g good quality dark chocolate, minimum 60% cocoa solids, chopped into small pieces

½ teaspoon ground cinnamon

500ml unsweetened almond milk

This luxurious drink combines the richness of dark chocolate with the warm spice of cinnamon for a real treat. Almond milk lends a sweet nuttiness.

Put the chocolate, cinnamon and almond milk into a pan and place over a medium-low heat. Whisk until the chocolate has melted and the milk is hot and frothy. Serve in large mugs.

5 WAYS WITH *flavoured water*

Although it is possibly the most important thing we consume, water intake is typically a low priority. Use your brain (75% of which is water) and replace caffeinated beverages and fruit juices – often avoided by patients during chemotherapy – with some of these refreshing, low sugar alternatives.

Sparkling water with cucumber and mint
Slice ¼ cucumber and divide between 2 glasses. Add 2 tbsp mint leaves and crush lightly with a spoon. Pour over ice-cold sparkling water and serve. 2 servings

Strawberry and basil water
Divide 100g halved, hulled strawberries and 2 tbsp basil leaves between 2 large glasses and crush lightly with a spoon. Half-fill the glasses with ice cubes and top up with still or sparkling water. Stir and serve. 2 servings

Citrus and rosemary water
Put 3 lightly bruised rosemary sprigs, 1 sliced orange and 1 sliced lemon in a large jug and top up with water until two-thirds full. Give it a good stir and allow to infuse for 30 minutes. Top up the jug with ice and serve. 4 servings

Apple and cinnamon infusion
Peel, core and slice 3 dessert apples. Toss 8 apple slices in a little lemon juice to stop them discolouring; set aside. Put the rest of the apples in a saucepan, pour on 550ml water and add a cinnamon stick. Bring to a simmer over a medium heat and simmer for 10 minutes, until the apples are soft and the water is nicely infused. Strain the hot water into mugs and serve topped with the remaining apple slices, as a winter warmer. 2 servings

Berry crush ice cubes
Take a handful of mixed berries, such as strawberries, blueberries and raspberries, and cut any larger fruit into small chunks. Distribute half of the berries equally among 1 or 2 ice-cube trays. Lightly crush the remaining fruit with a fork and divide among the trays. Squeeze over some lemon juice, top up with water and freeze for at least 2 hours. Add a few of the fruity ice cubes to a glass of still or sparkling water for a refreshing infusion.

Bibliography

Diet and breast cancer, understanding risks and benefits Thomson CA. Nutrition in Clinical Practice, Oct 2012, 27(5), pp. 636–50.

WHO, 2014 Cancer: Fact sheet N°297. Available from World Health Organization: who.int/mediacentre/factsheets/fs297/en

Modification in the diet can induce beneficial effects against breast cancer Aragón F, Perdigón G, de Moreno de LeBlanc A. World Journal of Clinical Oncology, Aug 2014, 5(3), pp.455–64.

Significant changes in dietary intake and supplement use after breast cancer diagnosis in a UK multicentre study Velentzis LS, Keshtgar MR, Woodside JV, Leathem AJ, Titcomb A, Perkins KA *et al*. Breast Cancer Research and Treatment, July 2011, 128(2), pp.473–82.

Multi-professional management of patients with breast cancer Lewis M, Davies I, Cooper J. Available from Cancer Research UK: cancerresearchuk.org

Breast and cervical cancer in 187 countries between 1980 and 2010: a systematic analysis Forouzanfar MH, Foreman KJ, Delossantos AM, Lozano R, Lopez AD, Murray CJ, Naghavi M. Lancet, Oct 2011, 378(9801), pp.1461–84.

The incidence of breast cancer: the global burden, public health considerations Forbes, JF. Seminars in Oncology, 1997, 24(1), pp.20–35.

Epidemiology of breast cancer: an environmental disease? Sasco AJ, APMIS, May 2001, 109, pp.321–32.

Cancer incidence in five continents. Perkins DM. International Agency for Research on Cancer, Scientific Publication 1997, 7, pp.1–1240.

Estimates of worldwide burden of cancer in 2008 GLOBOCAN 2008 International. Ferlay J, Shin HR, Bray F, Forman D, Mathers C, Parkin DM. Journal of Cancer, Dec 2010, 127, pp.2893–2917.

Adherence to the Mediterranean diet and risk of breast cancer The European prospective investigation into cancer and nutrition cohort study. Buckland G, Travier N, Cottet V *et al*. International Journal of Cancer, June 2013, 132(12), pp.2918–2927.

Diet and breast cancer: a systematic review Mourouti N, Kontogianni MD, Papavagelis C, Panagiotakos DB. International Journal of Food Sciences and Nutrition, Feb 2015, pp.1–42.

Food, nutrition, physical activity and the prevention of cancer: a global perspective Washington DC. World Cancer Research Fund, American Institute for Cancer Research (AICR). AICR, 2007.

Physical activity and risk of breast cancer overall and by hormone receptor status The European prospective investigation into cancer and nutrition. Steindorf K, Ritte R, Eomois PP, Lukanova A *et al*. International Journal of Cancer, April 2013, 132(7), pp.1667–78.

Physical activity and health: a report of the Surgeon General US Dept of Health and Human Services, Centers for Disease Control and Prevention, National Center for Chronic Disease Prevention and Health Promotion, 1996.

Body mass index and survival in women with breast cancer Systematic literature review and meta-analysis of 82 follow-up studies. Chan DS, Vieira AR, Aune D, Bandera EV, Greenwood DC, McTiernan A *et al*. Annals of Oncology, Oct 2014, 10, pp.1901–14.

Weight change in middle adulthood and breast cancer risk The EPIC-PANACEA study. Emaus MJ, Van Gils CH, Bakker MF, Bisschop CN *et al*. International Journal of Cancer, Dec 2014, 135(12), pp.2887–99.

Effect of obesity and other lifestyle factors on mortality in women with breast cancer Prospective Analysis of Case-control studies on Environmental factors and health (PACE) study group. Maso LD, Zucchett A, Talamini R, Serraino D, Stocco CF, Marina Vercelli *et al*. International Journal of Cancer, Nov 2008, 123(9), pp.2188-94.

Links between alcohol consumption and breast cancer: a look at the evidence Liu Y, Nguyen N, Colditz GA. Women's Health (London England), Jan 2015, 11(1), pp.65–77.

Alcohol consumption and breast cancer survival: a meta-analysis of cohort studies Gou YJ, Xie DX, Yang KH, Liu YL, Zhang JH, Li B, He XD. Asian Pacific Journal of Cancer Prevention, 2013, 14(8), pp.478–90.

Breast cancer survival in African American women: Is alcohol consumption a prognostic indicator? Paige A, McDonald PA, Williams R, Dawkins F, Adams-Campbell Ll. Cancer Causes & Control, Aug 2002, 13, pp.543–9.

Moderate alcohol consumption during adult life, drinking patterns and breast cancer risk Chen WY, Rosner B, Hankinson SE, Colditz GA, Willett WC. Journal of the American Medical Association, Nov 2011, 306, pp.1920–1

Useful websites

Case-control study of phytoestrogens and breast cancer Ingram D, Sanders K, Kolybaba M, Lopez D. Lancet, Oct 1997, 350, pp.990–4.

Urinary phytoestrogen excretion and breast cancer risk among Chinese women in Shanghai Dai Q, Franke AA, Jin F, Shu XO, Cluster LJ, Cheng J et al. Cancer Epidemiology Biomarkers and Prevention, Sept 2002, 11, pp.815–21.

The DietCompLyf study: a prospective cohort study of breast cancer survival and phytoestrogen consumption Swann R, Perkins KA, Velentzis LS, Ciria C, Dutton SJ, Dwek MV et al. Maturitas, July 2013, 75(3), pp.232–40.

Dietary lignan intakes in relation to survival among women with breast cancer: the Western New York exposures and breast cancer study McCann SE, Thompson LU, Nie J et al. Breast Cancer Research and Treatment, July 2010, 122, pp.229–35.

Soy food intake and breast cancer survival Shu XO, Zheng Y, Cai H et al. Journal of the American Medical Association, Dec 2009, 302, pp.2437–43.

Differential influence of dietary soy intake on the risk of breast cancer recurrence related to HER2 status Woo HD, Park KS, Ro J, Kim J. Nutrition and Cancer, Jan 2012, 64, pp.198–205.

Phytoestrogens and prevention of breast cancer: the contentious debate Bilal I, Chowdhury A, Davidson J, Whitehead S. World Journal of Clinical Oncology, Oct 2014, 5(4), pp.705–12.

Soy food consumption and breast cancer prognosis Cancer Epidemiology Biomarkers and Prevention. Caan BJ, Natarajan L, Parker B, Gold EB, Thomson C, Newman V et al. Feb 2011, 20(5), pp.854–8.

Intake of dairy products, calcium and vitamin D and risk of breast cancer Shin MH, Holmes MD, Hankinson SE, Wu K, Colditz GA, Willett WC. Journal of the National Cancer Institute, Sept 2002, 94(17), pp.1301–11.

Intakes of calcium and vitamin D and breast cancer risk in women Lin J, Manson JE, Lee IM, Cook NR, Buring JE, Zhang SM. Archives of International Medicine, May 2007, 167(10), pp.1050–9.

Major food sources of calories, added sugars and saturated fats and their contribution to essential nutrient intakes in the US diet Huth et al. Nutrition Journal 2013, 12, p116 www.nutritionj.com/content/12/1/116

Effects of dietary fatty acid composition from a high fat meal on satiety Kozimor A et al. Appetite, Oct 2013, 69, pp.39–45 www.ncbi.nlm.nih.gov/pubmed/23688821

Plasma free 25-hydroxyvitamin D, vitamin D binding protein, and risk of breast cancer The Nurses' Health Study II. Wang J, Eliassen H, Spiegelman D, Willett WC, Hankinson SE. Cancer Causes Control, April 2014, 25(7), pp.819–27

Consumption of Antioxidant-Rich Beverages and Risk for Breast Cancer in French Women Hirvonen T, Mennen LI, de Bree A, Castetbon K, Galan P, Bertrais S et al. Annals of Epidemiology, July 2006, 16, pp.503–8.

Post-diagnosis dietary factors and survival after invasive breast cancer Beasley JM, Newcomb PA, Trentham-Dietz A, Hampton JM, Andrew J. Bersch, Michael N et al. Breast Cancer Research and Treatment, Jan 2011, 128(1), pp.229–36.

Nutritional analysis All recipes were analysed using NetWISP nutritional software version 4, © 2006-2015 Tinuviel Software

Breast Cancer Care Information and support for anyone affected by breast cancer www.breastcancercare.org.uk

Breast Cancer.org Breast cancer awareness and information www.breastcancer.org

Breakthrough Breast Cancer Breast cancer research charity www.breakthrough.org.uk

National Cancer Institute US site offering information on breast cancer and treatment cancerwww.cancer.gov/cancertopics/types/breast

Cancer Research UK Charity raising funds for research into all forms of cancer www.cancerresearchuk.org

Dana-Farber Cancer Institute US cancer research organisation www.dana-farber.org/

British Nutrition Foundation Information and news of emerging food and nutrition related issues www.nutrition.org.uk/

Dr Susan Love Research Foundation US organisation providing information on breast cancer prevention, detection and treatment www.dslrf.org/breastcancer

Susan G Komen US charity funding breast cancer research and support ww5.komen.org/BreastCancer/AboutBreastCancer.html

World Cancer Research Fund International Continuous Update Project Report: diet, nutrition, physical activity and breast cancer survivors. www.wcrf.org/sites/default/files/Breast-Cancer-Survivors-2014-Report.pdf

Recipe analysis and further information www.westminster.ac.uk/breastcancercookbook www.ucl.ac.uk/breastcancercookbook www.royalfree.nhs.uk/breastcancercookbook

Index

Dedication

'I am grateful to all my breast cancer patients
who inspired me to do this book.'

M Keshtgar

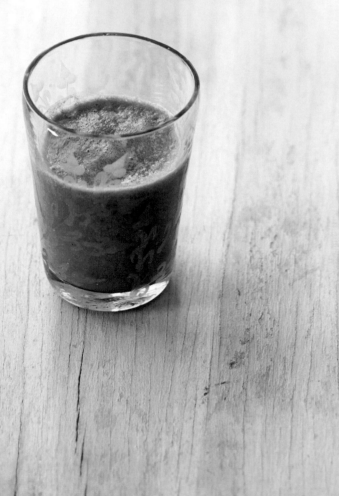

Jane O'Shea Publishing Consultant
Helen Lewis Creative Director
Janet Illsley Project Editor
Lucy Gowans Art Direction & Design
Jan Baldwin Photographer
Emily Jonzen Recipes & Food Styling
Rachel Dukes Props Styling
Vincent Smith, Tom Moore Production

Professor Mohammed Kestgar Faculty of Medical
Sciences, University College London, and Consultant
Breast Cancer Specialist, Royal Free London
Dr Claire Robertson Registered Nutritionist,
University of Westminster
Dr Miriam Dwek Reader, Group Leader
Breast Cancer Research Unit,
University of Westminster

First published in 2015 by
Quadrille Publishing Limited
www.quadrille.co.uk

Text © 2015 Mohammed Keshtgar
Recipes © 2015 Quadrille Publishing Limited
Photography © 2015 Jan Baldwin
Design and layout © 2015 Quadrille
Publishing Limited

Cataloguing in Publication Data:
a catalogue record for this book
is available from the British Library.

ISBN 978 184949 556 1

Printed in China